Lecture Notes: The Social B of M

The Queen Elizabeth Hospital
King's Lynn
NHS Trust

This book is dedicated to Jane, Euan and Ben, and to my mother, Val.

Lecture Notes

The Social Basis of Medicine

Andrew Russell

BA, MSc, DPhil
Senior Lecturer
Department of Anthropology/School of Medicine and Health
Durham University

WILEY-BLACKWELL

A John Wiley & Sons, Ltd., Publication

This edition first published 2009, © 2009 by Andrew Russell

Blackwell Publishing was acquired by John Wiley & Sons in February 2007. Blackwell's publishing program has been merged with Wiley's global Scientific, Technical and Medical business to form Wiley-Blackwell.

Registered office: John Wiley & Sons Ltd, The Atrium, Southern Gate, Chichester, West Sussex, PO19 8SQ, UK

Editorial offices: 9600 Garsington Road, Oxford, OX4 2DQ, UK
        The Atrium, Southern Gate, Chichester, West Sussex, PO19 8SQ, UK
        111 River Street, Hoboken, NJ 07030-5774, USA

For details of our global editorial offices, for customer services and for information about how to apply for permission to reuse the copyright material in this book please see our website at www.wiley.com/wiley-blackwell

Library of Congress Cataloging-in-Publication Data

Russell, Andrew, 1958–
   Lecture notes. The social basis of medicine / Andrew Russell.
      p. ; cm.
   Includes bibliographical references.
   ISBN 978-1-4051-3912-0
1. Social medicine. I. Title. II. Title: Social basis of medicine.
   [DNLM: 1. Social Medicine. WA 31 R961L 2009]
   RA418.R87 2009
   362.1–dc22
                              2008042542

ISBN: 978-1-4051-3912-0

A catalogue record for this book is available from the British Library.

Set in 8 on 12 pt Stone Serif by SNP Best-set Typesetter Ltd., Hong Kong

Printed in Singapore by Utopia Press Pte Ltd

1   2009

Contents

Preface

This book is written for medical students as well as recently graduated and practising doctors and other health professionals who wish to know more about and reflect on the social basis of medicine. This book aims to provide a readable and thought-provoking introduction to what is increasingly recognized as an area crucial to good medical practice. It is relevant to all doctors, not just those practising in community or public health settings.

The General Medical Council (GMC), in its path-breaking 'Tomorrow's Doctors', calls for medical education to 'foster the development of a caring, knowledgeable, competent and skilful medical graduate who broadly understands health and disease of the individual, the family and society, and who is able to benefit from subsequent medical education and adapt to future developments in practice', a graduate with 'respect for patients and colleagues that encompasses, without prejudice, diversity of background and opportunity, language, culture and way of life'. In other words, the doctor needs to have an approach that is more than biological, but encompasses the psychological and social aspects of medicine in both health care delivery and – increasingly importantly – health promotion. This biopsychosocial approach has come to be regarded as the 'gold standard' in the discipline, and is the foundation of the material contained in this book.

The education of doctors to practise integrated medicine and whole-person care requires a broad approach, involving not just the traditional basic medical sciences but other disciplines too. This book is unique in taking a multidisciplinary, 'human sciences' approach, introducing ideas and examples from a range of subjects, including medical sociology, medical anthropology, health psychology, health economics, the history of medicine, primary health care, public health and epidemiology, feminism, humanities, politics and economics. The object is not to teach medical students these subjects, but to show how the issues they raise can be applied to clinical and other contexts of medical practice. The book draws deeply on current research in this rapidly expanding field, with examples taken from the UK and around the world.

Chapter 1 introduces the biopsychosocial approach and situates medicine within the broader health system. Medicine is seen as both changing society (medicalization) and being changed by it (socialization). Chapter 2 looks at people's ideas about health, illness and how the body works, which can have profound effects on how they access health care and what types of health care they choose. The next three chapters look at the different sectors of health care within which health care takes place – the popular, professional and folk sectors. The coming together of doctors and patients in the consultation is the focus of Chapter 6.

Health and health care are not randomly distributed in any society, and the nature of health inequalities in the UK and globally is the subject of Chapter 7. The focus is on social class as a determinant of health inequalities. Chapter 8 looks at gender and ethnicity in a similar way. After this, we look at particular areas of health and health care in which the social basis of medicine is particularly prominent or important: in mental health, in dealing with disability, health promotion, chronic illness, death and dying, and in international health. The chapters are all designed to be read and worked on separately, or they can be followed in sequence. There is ample cross-referencing between chapters and to other books in the Lecture Notes series.

Unlike some areas of medical education, few aspects of socially-based medicine are factually cut and dried. Different opinions and theories exist concerning virtually all the topics covered. Rather than explicitly detailing the theories and the thinkers who created them, theory remains implicit in the text and the examples used. The book follows the style of other volumes in the Lecture Notes series by eschewing citations and footnotes. Instead, further readings at the end of each chapter direct you to the original sources from where many of the ideas expressed come, as well as to other useful books, journals and websites relevant to the topics covered. Case Studies give practical examples of the application of the issues raised to health and health care, while Points of View invite you to consider medically relevant questions arising from the issues covered. These are intended as discussion prompts rather than as questions that have a 'right' or 'wrong' answer, and should be useful for seminar and tutorial work.

The social and cultural field of medicine is fascinating, dynamic and rapidly changing. Comments on this edition and suggestions for future editions are welcome to ensure the social basis of medicine is represented in medical curricula with the most up-to-date ideas and information available.

Acknowledgements

I am grateful to the following people for their expert advice or for their assistance in formulating and discussing ideas: Gillian Bentley, David Chadwick, David Chappel, Louisa Ells, Victoria Gill, John Hamilton, Kate Hampshire, Cecil Helman, Pali Hungin, David Hunter, Marie Johnson, Ali Jones, Eileen Kaner, Sue Lewis, Jane Macnaughton, Sheena McDonald, John McLachlan, Ron Neville, Sarah Pearce, Tessa Pollard, Edwin Pugh, Jane Roberts, Tom Shakespeare, Simon Sinclair, Rosie Stacy, Helen Sykes, Mike White, Cathy Williamson, Nigel Wright as well as to tutors on the MBBS Phase I Medicine programme at Queen's Campus, Stockton, in particular Mwenza Blell, Lyn Brierley-Jones, Lauren Brooks, Serena Heckler, Emily Henderson, Steve Leech, Naz Iqbal and Alison Todd, and to members of the Medical Education and Medical Anthropology Research Groups at Durham not already mentioned above. Staff at Blackwell Publishing have been very helpful in seeing the book through to fruition, particularly Martin Sugden (who suggested the title), Hayley Salter, Laura Murphy and Vicki Donald, and their anonymous reviewers gave many useful suggestions for its improvement. Ruth Willats provided excellent copy editing services. Support for completing the book was provided by a fellowship from CETL-4HealthNE administered through the School of Health and Medicine at Durham University.

Material from many sources is included in this volume. The Author and Publisher have made every effort to contact all copyright holders to obtain their permission to reproduce copyright material. However, if any have been inadvertently overlooked, the Publisher will be pleased to make the necessary arrangements at the first opportunity. All UK Crown copyright material is reproduced with the permission of the Controller Office of Public Sector Information (OPSI).

Chapter 1

The social basis of medicine

No man is an island, entire of itself; every man is a piece of the continent, a part of the main. If a clod be washed away by the sea, Europe is the less, as well as if a promontory were, as well as if a manor of thy friend's or of thine own were. Any man's death diminishes me, because I am involved in mankind; and therefore never send to know for whom the bell tolls; it tolls for thee.

John Donne (1572–1631) *Meditation XVII* (extract)

Introduction

There is more to medicine than the basic sciences if one is to practise as a competent and humane physician. Effective patient care involves an appreciation not only of the biological but also of the psychological and social dimensions of every case. This biopsychosocial approach has become the 'gold standard' in medical practice and is the foundation of this book. It is fundamental to the practice of integrative medicine and whole-person care.

In order to practise using the biopsychosocial model, it is useful to view medicine as part of a wider health system. In some ways, the part medicine has to play, while vital, is small compared to what goes on in the three sectors of health care as a whole. Yet the influence of medicine in society is increasing, and the growing infiltration of medical knowledge and practice into domains that were previously not part of its remit is indicative of what is known as the medicalization of society. Conversely, medicine is imbued with the values of the society within which it is practised and is accountable to it. This is the socialization of medicine.

The biopsychosocial approach in clinical practice

Table 1.1 illustrates how the biopsychosocial approach can be used to understand the health problems of an individual or group. The three components of the biopsychosocial model of health and health care are the biological, the

Lecture Notes: *The Social Basis of Medicine*, 1st edition. By Andrew Russell. Published 2009 by Blackwell Publishing. ISBN: 978-1-4051-3912-0

Table 1.1 The biopsychosocial model.

BIO	PSYCHO	SOCIAL
Genetic factors	Loneliness	Poverty
Body system function	Self-esteem	Access to resources (e.g. healthy food)
(e.g. immune system)	Power and control	Living conditions (e.g. danger and stress at work or home)
		Discrimination

Table 1.2 The biomedical and biopsychosocial models compared.

Biomedical model	Biopsychosocial model
Body as biological	Body as biological and psychosocial
Biological processes separate from psychological and social processes	Biological, psychological and social processes intimately related
Disease or physical disorders can be explained by disturbances in physiological processes, e.g. injury, biochemical imbalances, infections	Illness can be explained by challenges to the whole person, a combination of biological, psychological and social factors
Disease requires specific treatment	Person requires individual treatment
Emphasis on cure	Emphasis on care

psychological and the social. They interact to affect the health of the individual or group. In any health care activity, it is necessary to take all three into account if care is to be provided that is sensitive to the 'whole person'. Of the three components, this book focuses on the social and psychological. Taking a psychological and social view not only assists our understanding of patients, it is also invaluable in working effectively with other members of the health team, and in appreciating the social, cultural and behavioural determinants of health and disease in general.

One way of conceptualizing the whole person in a biopsychosocial way is by means of a hierarchy of systems.

Hierarchy of systems in the biopsychosocial model

Society
Culture
Community
Family
Person
Organs/organ systems
Tissues
Cells
Genes
Molecules

These ten systems are interrelated, in that an individual 'case' will encapsulate all of them. By 'society' what is meant is the structure and organization of everyday life, which corresponds also to a definition of the 'social', and by culture we mean the beliefs, attitudes and behaviours of groups and individuals, which correspond to a definition of 'cultural'. In focusing on the psychological and social aspects of the model, this book focuses on the hierarchy from 'person' upwards.

The biopsychosocial model of health and illness is often contrasted with the biomedical model of disease (Table 1.2).

Doctors are taught during their training to single out disease as an organic pathology (diagnosis) from the story ('history') of the illness experience of the sick. Because biomedicine is unique in that it grounds its knowledge in materialism (in a realm of 'facts'), it has a tendency to detach the facts of bodily function and disease from their social and cultural context. A sick person, then, may find themselves reconstrued as a body, a case, a patient or a cadaver, rather than as a 'person'. However, the distinction between the biomedical and biopsychosocial approaches is confusing, since few good doctors use only a biomedical approach in modern medicine. What the biopsychosocial approach does is expand the biomedical view by adding psychological and social factors to biological ones as needful of consideration.

Integrative medicine and whole-person care

The biopsychosocial approach requires the practice of what is known as integrative medicine. Such an approach combines knowledge from the body systems and the social and behavioural systems that is used in an integrated way, for the purpose of what is known as 'whole-person care'. For whole-person care to be effective, it requires not only that the medical practitioner integrates knowledge and information from diverse sources, but also that the medical services operate in an integrated manner with other health and social services – the health care team.

There are three main reasons why we need to understand how the psychosocial factors operate. First, practising medicine requires that we understand the social and cultural backgrounds of the patients we serve as well as those of their carers, friends and families. People's beliefs and practices with regard to health and illness vary widely, both within and between cultures. Taking these things into account is essential for *patient-centred* medicine, whether it is aimed at promoting good health or delivering effective health care.

Second, we need to understand the social and cultural basis of our own backgrounds and professional practice, as well as those of colleagues in other health care professions. This is the approach of the *reflective practitioner*, another gold standard of clinical practice. The beliefs and practices of the lay public may well differ from those of the health care professions, and the health care professions differ in turn in their approaches and philosophies.

Third, social, cultural and psychological factors contribute to explaining why 'health' is not evenly distributed in a particular locality, region, nation or the world in general. It is important that we take *health inequalities* into account if we are to apportion health care equitably and to devise solutions in both clinical and public health medicine that are of optimum benefit to those that need them.

Case study: The need for 'whole-person care'

Entering your general practice one morning, you spot Mel, a 16-year-old girl with cystic fibrosis. Her eyes are puffy and it looks like she has recently been crying. She is overweight and seems to be inadequately dressed for the time of year. When you invite her into your consulting room she comes in, sits down and promptly bursts into tears. Her parents have been rowing, she says, and this morning her stepfather walked out. You talk through the difficulties she has been having and ask her if there is anything else that may be bothering her.

'Yes', she says, 'I think I'm pregnant.'

How would a biopsychosocial approach help in dealing with Mel's problems?

What is a health system?

A health system may be defined as the sum total of the institutions and practices through which individuals, families, communities and society maintain and improve health and deal with ill health.

The components of a health system

- Institutions
  - formal
  - informal
- Activities
  - clinical practices
  - non-clinical practices
- Skills
- Knowledge
- Beliefs and attitudes

In the UK the National Health Service (NHS) is the major formal institution (it is the largest single employer in the UK) with responsibility for delivering health to the nation. An example of an informal institution is the household, an important venue for health-seeking behaviour among the general population. Clinical practice takes place in a variety of settings, but even more varied are the places in which non-clinical practices that affect health may be found. The skills required for a health system to function effectively are unevenly distributed within it. In general practice within the UK, for example, practice nurses are not allowed to prescribe drugs, but nurse practitioners can. Knowledge about health and illness is similarly unequally distributed. Finally, beliefs and attitudes permeate every aspect of health and health care. These institutions, practices, knowledge and beliefs are all interconnected. They cannot be understood in isolation from other aspects of society (e.g. social, religious, political and economic organization). In accordance with UK law, for example, particular kinds of knowledge and practice are concentrated in certain institutions (such as hospitals or acupuncture clinics) and not in others. The growth of interest and activities concerned with health in modern society has led to a meteoric expansion of organizations concerned with health and health care delivery.

The health system we have not only creates institutions, skills and knowledge within society, it also reflects the priorities and prejudices of society – for example, in our treatment of the elderly, mental as opposed to physical health care, and the division of labour by sex, class and ethnicity.

The three sectors of health care	
Popular	Informal
Folk		
Professional	Formal

Most health care takes place in the *popular sector*, often without reference to a folk or professional healer. Estimates vary, but between 70% and 90% of all health care takes place in this sector, in both western and non-western societies. The popular sector is the focus of Chapter 3.

The *folk sector* is characterized in the UK by different types of complementary or alternative medicine. Some of these may also be 'professional' (e.g. homeopathy) or 'professionalizing'. In India, for example, Ayurvedic medicine, which in the UK is generally regarded as a folk or alternative tradition, is part of mainstream medicine. In fact, students on medical courses in India often study a common foundation course before going on to specialize in either Ayurvedic or western biomedical (or allopathic) medicine. The folk sector is the subject matter of Chapter 5.

The *professional sector* includes all medical and paramedical groups and professionals. Each group has a different history and culture, reflected in different perceptions of health and ill health, forms of treatment, defined areas of competence, internal hierarchy, technical jargon and professional organizations. The professional sector is examined in Chapter 4.

These three sectors interact, both internally and with other systems, including the religious, economic and political systems operating in any society. Where these different institutions interact, *medical pluralism* exists. People's decision-making with regard to different types of therapy – their health-seeking behaviour – is discussed in Chapter 2.

The three sectors of health care

Three types of institutional arrangements for providing health care can be identified within any society, along a spectrum from informal to formal.

The medicalization of society

The relationship between the three sectors is not static. In particular, the 'professional' sector, represented by modern medical practice, is increasingly pervasive in people's lives (the 'popular' sector).

This increased influence is known as the medicalization of society, and resistance to it is marked by demedicalization. Probably what is happening is that the 'popular' and 'professional' sectors are becoming more integrated, with the medicalization of society paralleled by an increasing socialization of medicine.

What is medicalization?

The process of defining an increasing number of life's problems as medical problems.

There are many areas of life in which medicine plays an increasingly prominent role; these include ageing, childbirth, alcohol and food consumption, and childhood behaviour. At the same time, medicine retains, or seeks to retain, absolute control over certain technical procedures, including prescribing, hysterectomy and abortion. There has also been an expansion of what in medicine is deemed relevant to the good practice of life, e.g. doctors being asked to comment as 'expert witnesses' in court cases on the mental state of defendants. This might be seen as the 'medicalization of deviance', where what were previously regarded as moral or social problems move into the medical domain (i.e. from 'bad' to 'sad'/'mad'). The increasing medicalization of society is often viewed negatively, but there are times when medicalizing behaviour as illness may be positive if it means that some form of treatment can be offered.

Women and children are particularly subject to medicalization. Areas in which medicalization can be observed for women include childbirth, menstruation and menstrual irregularities, new reproductive technologies (e.g. infertility treatments), new contraceptive technologies, premenstrual syndrome and hormone replacement therapy (HRT) during the menopause. Children are also likely to spend more time with health professionals, and to have far more monitoring, than they did in the past. Some children will be ascribed, and given treatments for, conditions previously undescribed or that are disputed, such as Attention Deficit Disorder (ADD) or Attention Deficit and Hyperactivity Disorder (ADHD).

Medicalization is marked by increasing

- Levels of pharmaceutical consumption.
- Use of other medical technologies.
- Frequency of visits to medical settings.
- Range and extent of medical services.
- Risk of iatrogenic diseases.
- Influence of medicine in previously non-medical domains.
- Levels of health surveillance.
- Media coverage of health and medical matters.
- Risk of iatrogenic diseases.

Increasing levels of pharmaceutical consumption

In any 24-hour period, about half the adult population of the UK are likely to consume a medically prescribed chemical. There is an increasing range of 'pills to pop', sometimes to treat problems that were previously regarded as non-medical (e.g. HRT for menopausal symptoms). If we add the products available without the need for prescription, medicalization through increased use of pharmaceutical products appears even more intense. The term 'cosmetic neurology' has been used to describe the use of drugs by otherwise healthy people to manipulate mood, memory, concentration, libido, capacity to learn and general ability to cope.

Increasing use of other medical technologies

As well as pharmaceuticals, there has been a tremendous growth in other types of medical technology. For example, there are increasing numbers of aids for disabled people. More and more people are depending on medical technology of various kinds (e.g. asthma 'puffers' and nebulizers, contraceptive implants, kidney dialysis machines, oxygen cylinders, cardiac pacemakers, life-support machines). Through such means, the half-human, half-machine 'cyborg' of science fiction comes closer to reality.

Increasing frequency of visits to medical settings

In the UK, in 1900 99% of births took place in the home. Eighty years later, this figure had reversed to 99% of births taking place in hospital. At the other end of life, increasing numbers of us are dying in hospital (see Chapter 13).

Increasing range and extent of medical services

The range and extent of medical services are expanding. New specialisms have developed, among them occupational therapy, geriatric medicine and palliative care. The NHS is now the largest single employer in the UK with over one million employees and is one of the largest employers in the world. In fact, in just about every country in the world, the number of people working in the health field is growing.

Increasing influence of medicine in previously non-medical domains

Doctors are expected to report to the authorities all diseases that carry the risk of mass infection, but also some conditions that don't (e.g. suicide attempts, gunshot wounds). New alliances – for example, between medicine and social workers, police, prison service, local authorities and other institutions that are concerned not only with welfare but also social control – are being formed. Medicine is infiltrating health and social care pathways that might previously have been outside its domain, in the provision of 'care in the community' for example, and in the work of 'health care teams'. The NHS is incorporating new areas into its remit, such as the increasing involvement of complementary practitioners in NHS-funded care. Doctors are also incorporating skills from other practitioners into their working methods, such as the use of counselling skills to deal with personal and social (rather than 'health') problems.

Doctors have also been at the forefront of various forms of social action (e.g. smoke free legislation). As well as their use by 'expert witnesses' in jury trials and inquests, medical evidence and practice (particularly in the field of public health) are used to advance arguments and causes – e.g. the fluoridation of water supplies.

While medicine obviously desires its self-perpetuation, the strengthening and (perhaps) enlargement of its sphere of influence, much of the authority from which medicine derives its power comes from the faith and trust the general public place in it (see below).

Increasing levels of health surveillance

Linked with the growing power of medicine is the rise in health surveillance as an increasingly normal part of everyday life in the West – another example of medicalization in action. Most women will, at some time, be asked when they last had a cervical smear test. Men similarly are under increasing surveillance for diseases such as prostate and testicular cancer. Babies and young children are the subject of numerous checks by health visitors, some of them in the home. More genetic tests (e.g. for breast cancer), and prenatal screening procedures (e.g. for Down's syndrome and spina bifida), may serve to heighten tension and anxiety among people who are the object of such tests.

Increasing media coverage of health and medical matters

Coverage of health and medicine in the media (magazines, newspapers, TV, etc.) reflects a growing interest in health issues among the general public, which cannot be attributed to 'media hype' alone. The public are more likely to expect and bring pressure for their GP to 'do something' (i.e. offer some kind of medical intervention). Despite the recent scandals concerning mortality rates in the Bristol Royal Infirmary child cardiac unit, the case of Harold Shipman, a GP estimated to have been responsible for the deaths of at least 250 of his elderly patients, and the retention of body parts at Alder Hey hospital, public confidence and faith in medical science remain strong – perhaps because in many spheres it is seen as the 'only hope'. This trend may be linked to the increasing secularization (i.e. decline in the influence of religion) in many sectors of society.

Increasing risk of iatrogenic diseases

With the growth of medicine, there are more examples of diseases in society that are caused by medical interventions themselves (so-called iatrogenic diseases). Antibiotic-resistant bacteria, for example, are the result of overuse and misuse of antibiotics in the treatment of infections.

Medicalization can be explained in the following ways

- Increasing medical knowledge
- Redefinition of social problems as medical problems
- Developments in medical technology (e.g. disease prevention, treatments and investigative procedures).
- Advent of new diseases and medical research attempting to combat them
- Public pressure.

Increasing medical knowledge

The ability of doctors to intervene in areas that were once beyond their competence – e.g. psychotropic drugs for mental illness, plastic surgery, sterilization, sleeping pills, appetite suppressants, anti-impotence drugs, sex-change procedures, abortions, 'triple therapy' for *Helicobacter pylori* infection (associated with duodenal ulcers, previously a largely chronic condition), 'new genetics' and genetic counselling.

Redefinition of social problems as medical problems – some examples

A drunkard	An alcoholic
Shell shock	Post-traumatic stress disorder
Child sex offender	Paedophile
Naughty child	Child with ADHD
Overweight	Obese
Unhappy	Depressed
Sleeplessness	Insomnia
'Time of life'	Menopause

Developments in medical technology

There are new preventive areas in which health professionals intervene – e.g. vaccinations and immunisations (for polio, MMR, whooping cough); vitamin pills and supplements; antenatal and postnatal classes; postnatal visits and check-ups by health visitors.

Increasing technological sophistication, combined with the 'technological imperative' (i.e. to intervene if you have the technology to do so), increases the likelihood of medical intervention. Examples include amniocentesis, CAT scans, blood tests, x-rays and surgical procedures such as transplants. Some of this new technology has amazing effects on individual longevity and quality of life (although is problematized in the public mind by the possibility of iatrogenesis – see above). With these evermore sophisticated techniques, people's reliance on medical 'experts' increases. This trend is likely to increase with the growth of 'new genetics'.

Advent of 'new' diseases and medical research to overcome them in the past 20 years – examples

HIV/AIDS
BSE (bovine spongiform encephalopathy or 'mad cow' disease)
SARS (severe acute respiratory syndrome)
Ebola virus
RSI (repetitive strain injury)
Chronic fatigue syndrome (myalgic encephalomyelitis, ME)

Pressure from public

While the media may have a role to play in increasing the concern, the high-profile coverage of health issues on TV and in magazines and newspapers is a reflection of greater interest in, and expectations regarding, health among the general public. People are taking more responsibility for their health (or are expected to do so according to various health promotion messages). For example, more people are doing their own research prior to visiting a doctor, on the internet and elsewhere, and are demanding more medical investigations and interventions. The increasing complexity and mobility of modern society means that older forms of social support (family or friends and neighbours) are not always readily available, and hence the likelihood of using medical services increases. With increased knowledge about health risks and lack of knowledge about what to do about them, perhaps people have become subtly socialized into believing themselves to be more vulnerable and needful of doctors than they were in the past.

Demedicalization

More recently there has been a movement against medicalization. This has generally been driven by patients voicing their rights as consumers, but it has also been supported by many members of the health professions.

Examples of demedicalization

- Home births and low-intervention hospital births
- Over-the-counter medicines
- Growth in complementary therapies
- Non-compliance with treatment

Home births and low-intervention hospital births

While in the 1980s the figure for home births stood at 1% in the UK, by the end of the 1990s this had increased to 2.2%. This trend reflects something of a backlash against the medicalization of pregnancy. Pregnancy, it is argued, is a natural, personal experience, not the unnatural, technical procedure it has become in hospital settings. Hospitals have responded by providing more low-technology 'birthing suites', which offer mothers and their carers an environment more like a comfortable home than a hospital. Much of the pressure for these changes has come from midwives based either in the community or hospital setting.

Over-the-counter medicines

The increasing number of pharmaceuticals available over the counter (OTC) at pharmacies, supermarkets and other shops is also an indication of demedicalization. Drugs that were once only available with a GP prescription (e.g. Canesten cream for vaginal thrush; emergency contraception – the 'morning-after' pill) can now be bought in a pharmacy.

Growth in complementary therapies

The current interest in complementary therapies in the UK reflects people's increased interest in health in general, but also their desire to find solutions that are more 'natural', less invasive and more holistic than the perceived offerings of the medical profession.

Non-compliance with treatment

There is evidence that despite the increasing levels of medicalization and surveillance, there is a great deal of non-compliance in participation and treatment. In other words, medicalization is not necessarily as widespread or as successful as might at first be thought. However, it remains a pervasive influence in society and one that must be taken into account in understanding people's perceptions of medicine in general (e.g. magical, mechanistic, risky) and doctors in particular, and in order to practise forms of medicine that are sensitive to these perceptions – in other words, to be a good doctor.

The socialization of medicine

While medicine has a growing influence in society, it also reflects and responds to the influences of the society in which it operates.

Examples of the socialization of medicine

- Roles and accountability within the NHS
- The clinical consultation
- The inverse care law
- Social medicine and community medicine

Roles and accountability within the NHS

In Chapter 4 we shall see how the roles of men and women are reproduced in the distribution of jobs in the NHS. The trend towards accountability in medicine reflects a more general shift in the way in which professionals are viewed and treated by society – the rise of 'audit culture' and what might be thought of as the greater surveillance of medicine by society.

The clinical consultation

Medicine is also, inevitably, socialized by the clinical encounter. A patient-centred approach requires that doctors take the social and cultural backgrounds of their patients into account when working with them and their problems. The social basis of medicine as reflected in the consultation is covered in Chapter 6.

The inverse care law

Another way in which medicine reflects society is in the distribution of health care services within and between communities. Julian Tudor Hart, a GP working in South Wales in 1971, coined the term 'inverse care law' to describe how health care is unevenly distributed, with those most in need receiving the least. Since then a major public health concern has been the recognition and rectification of such inequality. This forms the subject matter of Chapter 7.

Social medicine and community medicine

The importance of the social context of medicine is recognized by the development of what has become known as 'social medicine' and 'community medicine'. Some specialities, such as palliative care, are particularly involved in practising forms of social medicine. Another indicator of the broader interests of modern medicine is the growth in the medical humanities movement, with its interest in the representation of medicine in the arts and humanities, and the application of these disciplines (such as literature, philosophy and the arts) in medicine. To an increasing extent, all branches of medicine are forms of 'social medicine'.

Summary

- The biopsychosocial approach is the 'gold standard' of modern medical practice and requires an understanding of the biological, psychological and social aspects of health and illness.
- Biopsychosocial medicine is the foundation of 'patient-centred' care, and of the 'whole-person' approach to the clinical consultation.
- It is important for doctors to understand the social basis of their own work and professional culture as part of a much larger and more complex health system.
- The health system is made up of three sectors – lay, folk and professional.
- Medicine as a profession plays an important and growing role in the life of the public (the 'medicalization of society').
- There are moves to reduce the pervasiveness of medicine ('demedicalization').
- Medicine is subject to the influence of the society of which it is a part (the 'socialization of medicine').
- Health and health care are not equally distributed within society, and social and psychological factors contribute to the inequalities in health that doctors must deal with on a daily basis.
- To an increasing extent, all branches of medicine are forms of social medicine.

Further reading

Alder, B. et al. (2004) *Psychology and Sociology Applied to Medicine: an Illustrated Colour Text* (2nd edn.). Edinburgh: Churchill Livingstone.

Engel, G. (1977) The need for a new medical model: a challenge for biomedicine. *Science*, **196**: 129–36.

General Medical Council (2003) *Tomorrow's Doctors: Recommendations on Undergraduate Medical Education*. London: General Medical Council.

Helman, C. (2007) *Culture, Health and Illness* (5th edn.). London: Hodder Arnold.

Moon, G. and Gillespie, R. (eds) (1995) *Society and Health: an Introduction to Social Science for Health Professionals*. London: Routledge.

Ogden, J. (2004) *Health Psychology: a Textbook* (3rd edn.). Maidenhead: Open University Press.

Sarafino, E. P. (2006) *Health Psychology: Biopsychosocial Interactions* (5th edn.). New York: Wiley.

Scambler, G. (2003) *Sociology as Applied to Medicine* (5th edn.). Edinburgh: Saunders.

Seale, C. (1994) Health and healing in an age of science. In C. Seale and S. Pattison (eds.) *Medical Knowledge: Doubt and Certainty*. Milton Keynes: Open University Press.

Senior, M. with B. Viveash (1998) *Health and Illness*. Basingstoke: Macmillan.

Taylor, R. J. et al. (2003) *Health and Illness in the Community*. Oxford: Oxford University Press.

Chapter 2

Beliefs about health, ill health and the body

Introduction

There are many ways in which people's beliefs, theories and knowledge impact on the prevalence, perceptions and presentation of health and disease. In addition, differences in concepts of health and ill health, and people's perceptions of how the body works, are important. We tend to use the terminology denoting health and ill health rather loosely in the English language. Yet these terms may have profoundly different meanings for different people, affecting their attitudes towards health and illness and the likelihood and manner of their seeking prevention or treatment of ill health. It is important that doctors consider the meanings that patients convey by the use of certain words such as health and illness in order to understand better their motivations and expectations, so that doctors can provide better patient-centred care. Similarly, people's beliefs about the body affect how they describe it in clinical consultations. Certain illnesses, as well as certain parts of the body, may be given negative attributes or be the subject of shame or embarrassment. Such emotions contribute to a sense of stigma about these illnesses or body parts.

Lecture Notes: *The Social Basis of Medicine*, 1st edition. By Andrew Russell. Published 2009 by Blackwell Publishing. ISBN: 978-1-4051-3912-0

> **This chapter covers the following topics**
>
> What is health?
> What is ill health? Disease, illness and sickness
> Explanations of ill health
> Labelling and stigma
> The body

What is health?

Health is a concept that is used pretty much unthinkingly by everyone. However, if people are asked to define it, the definitions they come up with are often surprisingly diverse. Rather than an absolute term in opposition to illness, health is better viewed as part of a continuum between death and optimal wellness (Figure 2.1). Often health and illness overlap. Many people, and particularly those suffering from a chronic condition, may exhibit signs of ill health, but nevertheless insist they are 'healthy for all that'.

People's perceptions of health will affect whether, and if so how, they access and use medical services.

Dimensions of health

There are three dimensions of health which are worth considering separately for what they tell

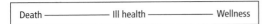

Death ——————— Ill health ——————— Wellness

Figure 2.1 The wellness–death continuum.

us about perceptions of health: these are the physical, mental and social. In all three, 'What is health?' is linked to what is perceived as 'normal'. Ideas of 'normality' vary quite markedly among groups and individuals.

Physical health

If we consider the body as a machine, then a combination of normal appearance, anatomical structure and physiological functioning is indicative of good health. However, what is regarded as 'normal' is linked to various factors.

Factors affecting what is regarded as 'normal' in physical health

- Age
- Social status
- Gender
- Geography
- Disability

Age

Telephone conversation from general practice:

'Mr Jones?'

'Aye.'

'You asked me to ring you to discuss a problem you've been having. What seems to be the matter?'

'Well, it's like this, I'm visiting the area and since I've been here I've been having trouble lifting things – for example, I couldn't lift the suitcase onto the bed. I feel all weak.'

'I think you should come in to see me immediately. Let me take a few details about you. What did you say your name was?'

'Jones. George Jones.'

'And what's your age, please, Mr Jones?'

'Ninety-four last February.'

Why is this exchange amusing? Our amusement lies in the degree to which we all share assumptions about what it is 'normal' for a 94-year-old to be able do.

Social status

Expectations of physical health are associated with social status (which is partly linked to class, see Chapter 7). As well as individuals of high social status having greater expectations concerning their health, we also expect our leaders and others in positions of power to demonstrate high levels of health and fitness. Women and men who fulfil the highest ideals of physical prowess are given titles, crowns or medals such as 'Miss World', 'Mr Universe', 'World Champion'.

Gender

Women and men differ in terms of having what is regarded as 'normal' physical health. Body-building illustrates this phenomenon. While opinions are changing and there are now contests for both sexes, female body-builders are generally regarded as 'abnormal' compared with male body-builders.

Geography

Obesity varies markedly in different parts of the world, and there is evidence that people become 'accustomed' to particular levels of obesity in their own society. 'Normal' body weight and size in the UK have been increasing over the years, as reflected in changing clothing sizes in shops and obesity in young adults. Under-nourishment may also come to be regarded as 'normal' in certain contexts (e.g. among fashion models).

'Normal' levels of fitness can also vary markedly both between societies and between groups within societies. In rural Nepal, for example, 'normal' agricultural work may involve carrying loads of up to 80 kg in a basket supported by a strap around the forehead. Such loads would cripple a typical western office worker.

The natural history of disease in particular places can also affect what is regarded as normal health. Napoleon Bonaparte called Egypt 'the land of menstruating men' because of the high levels of blood in the urine of its inhabitants caused by schistosomiasis, a parasitical infection (also called bilharzia). In parts of rural Egypt where schistosomiasis is rife, young boys can sometimes be seen jumping in the red urine of those who have the disease in a vain attempt to 'catch' what is considered a 'normal' condition.

Disability

Physical incapacity can also be considered 'normal' by those who have it, so that some groups come to reject the label 'disabled' and regard themselves as 'differently abled'. (This is dealt with in more depth in Chapter 10.)

Mental health

Mental health even more than physical health is a problematic concept to define. This is because it is based on the inner psychological state of the individual or group, which can only be indirectly appraised through the study of behaviour and communication, both verbal and non-verbal. The following definitions of mental health have been suggested:

Definitions of Mental Health

The capacity to live in a resourceful and fulfilling manner, having the resilience to deal with the challenges and obstacles which life presents
(Leeds University Ahead 4 Health)

Positive mental health is about:
- feeling in control
- being able to make rational decisions
- being in touch with our feelings
- being able to form positive relationships
- feeling good about ourselves
- knowing how to look after ourselves
(Oxford Brookes University Student Services)

Mental health can be further subdivided into intellectual health and emotional health. The two appear to work in tandem, so that good intellectual health is generally associated with emotional

health and vice versa, perhaps because those in possession of intellectual resources are better able to manage their emotions in positive and constructive ways. However, there are many exceptions to this rule. The term 'emotional intelligence' is now used in education to describe the bringing together of these two strands in the promotion of mental health in young people and adults. What is regarded as 'normal' mental health is highly dependent on social context (see Chapter 9).

Social health

This component of health involves the types, number and quality of relationships we have. These relationships can involve husband, wife, partner, brother, sister, uncle, aunt, cousin, friend, employer, employee, patient, caregiver, coach, team member, neighbour, etc.

There are various ways of measuring social health, through the analysis of networks and social capital. Some of these are presented in Chapter 3.

Models of Health

Negative models of health and their clinical implications

The medical view of health (see Table 2.1) is regarded as 'negative' because it is based on what is *not* present (i.e. disease, illness and injury) and says nothing about what is present when health is good. This can lead to a mismatch between patient and health care provider, if the patient is looking for health in which certain positive states can be identified, while the doctor is attempting to diagnose and deal with the physical manifestation of ill health that has been presented. However, not all patients are necessarily looking for more than something being fixed (physical health; see above), and in some cases the doctor may have to suggest that a more positive view of health is appropriate.

The medical model of health is ultimately impossible because there are few people who could claim to have their full body functions and a total absence of any disease, illness or infirmity. In Peckham, south London, in the 1920s, for example, a study for a health centre found that

Table 2.1 Three models of health.

Model	Definition	Comments
Medical	Health = absence of disease, illness and injury	= 'negative' view
Social sciences/Functional	Health = the ability to function in normal social roles	What defines a 'normal social role' and what of the 'sick role'?
Idealist	Health = a state of complete physical, mental and social well-being, and not merely the absence of disease or infirmity	= World Health Organization (WHO)'s definition; biopsychosocial; 'positive' view

Numerous other models of health have been identified. One is the idea of 'health as fitness'; another is the idea of health as 'social relationships' – the ability to make and maintain relationships with people; a third is the idea of 'health as potential', the degree to which an individual has made full use of opportunities and copes with adversity.

only 9% of people in what was then considered to be a relatively comfortable suburb, without extremes of wealth or poverty, were free of some kind of clinical disorder. In the medical mind, everyone is latently unhealthy. This raises the potential of labelling people as unhealthy who would disagree with such a diagnosis (see below).

Positive models of health and their clinical implications

The WHO's definition of health (see Table 2.1), with its focus on physical, mental and social well-being, is 'positive' because it is concerned not only with being disease-free but also with what happens in this state, and takes the multidimensional view that health is more than a question of biology. It can thus be compared with the biopsychosocial approach in clinical practice (discussed in Chapter 1). However, like the medical model, the WHO's definition is ultimately an unattainable (i.e. an 'ideal') view of health and has been criticized for this reason. However, like the biopsychosocial model it supports a holistic approach to practice, one based on whole-person care.

Case study: Negative and positive models of health in a clinical context

Mrs Wright visits her GP with a history of headaches, which may be migraine. She says she feels well otherwise, although she has been under a lot of stress at work (she works at a nearby airport as a check-in agent). She says: *'If only I could get rid of these headaches, I'd be healthy.'*

Joe Collins, age 48, visits his GP complaining of snoring.
'It's keeping my wife awake at night. I even think it's been waking me up recently. We're getting tetchy with each other.'

In each case, identify the model of health that is being exhibited, and how the GP might best handle the situation.

Points of view: Are these people healthy?

The purpose of this exercise is to explore your assumptions and expectations of health. Consider the four cases below and, using the chart, mark with a tick or a cross whether you think the person is healthy according to the three models of health presented in Table 2.1.

	Selma	Geronimo	Gavin	Joleyn
Medical				
Social Sciences				
Idealist				

Selma is a 38-year-old Anglo-Indian who lives in north London. She had a good job as a social worker with her local borough council until, on her way to visit a client, she was involved in a serious car accident, when a vehicle travelling in the opposite direction forced her off the road and into a lamp-post. She is now paraplegic, lacking the use of her legs and lower torso. She lives in a specially designed flat and has been on her own since her husband left her without warning following her accident. Yet she feels content, has a good circle of friends and still concerns herself with the needs and aspirations of those less well off than herself. She has become something of a champion for disabled rights, and writes articles for the press and magazines. She receives help from health and social services, paid for by the state, and has a good income from interest earned from the compensation she received from the insurers of the driver who caused the accident and supplementary income from her writing.

Geronimo is a 21-year-old white male from a reasonably well-off, middle-class background in the Midlands. He has been estranged from his parents since he was 17 due to disagreements over his politics and lifestyle, and does not currently have a permanent address, sleeping most nights on the floors of friends' 'squats', or in a tent or caravan with his dog, Moser. He had a brush with the law during the time of the G8 world leaders' summit in Gleneagles, Scotland, when protestors against globalization and environmental degradation were arrested but subsequently released without charge. In common with most of his friends, Geronimo has never had a full-time job, but deals in 'soft' drugs in a small way in order to supplement his social security benefit. Although he smokes 'roll-ups', he is in good physical shape, partly because of the regular exercise he takes walking Moser, and cuts a striking figure with his dreadlocks and grey trench coat open to the elements.

Gavin is a 52-year-old a white male originally from Scotland, who has done well as a businessman trading in ceramic ornaments. He is married with two sons, both of whom are at university. He lives in a luxurious detached house in a prosperous suburb of Chester. He has a good circle of friends and business acquaintances, plays two rounds of golf every week and is an active member of the local branch of the Conservative Party. He enjoys the trappings of his wealth – he has a good 'wine cellar' and drinks two or three glasses of wine a day, often followed by a malt whisky 'nightcap'. He also enjoys smoking the occasional cigar when he is socializing. He tries to keep his weight down since he cares about his appearance but has noticed a bit of a 'spare tyre' forming over the past couple of years. There has been a downturn in the market recently and this has halted his ambitious plans for expansion. Frustrated easily, Gavin is sometimes prone to fits of temper. Twice recently he has slapped his wife in the face with the back of his hand.

Joleyn is a 20-year-old black female whose parents are originally from Jamaica. She lives in a fourth floor council flat in Birmingham with her son Ben, who is three years old. The wallpaper is peeling because of damp in one of the rooms, and the lifts often don't work, but Joleyn is determined to make the best of things because she feels lucky to have a roof over her head. When she was five she spent nine weeks in care following the breakdown of her parents' relationship. Her father returned to Jamaica and has had no further contact with her; her mother began a new relationship but the stepfather and Joleyn have never seen 'eye to eye'. Her pregnancy was something of a mistake and led to a rift with her mother and stepfather which has been slow to heal, although Joleyn has never regretted having Ben. Living in her new accommodation has brought Joleyn into contact with Denise, who lives in the flat below and also has a small child. The two women share childcare so that Joleyn can work as a cleaner to supplement her social security benefit. Joleyn has recently met a man who she feels is 'different from the rest' and is likely to be a 'good bet' for her and Ben.

Factors affecting consumers' perspectives on health

In studies of people's beliefs about health, various age, class and gender differences have been found in the models of health people use.

Age

Young men in particular have been observed to have a 'health as fitness' model. Older people tend to start using the 'functional' model of health.

Class

In the UK, the 'functional' model tends to be associated with the lower social classes while the idealist model is associated with the middle and upper classes.

Gender

Women are more likely to be found using a 'health as social relationships' model – health as having good relationships with family and children, having patience with and enjoying them.

These differences are important clinically because they affect people's perceptions of their own and other people's health and ill-health, and the '*health-seeking behaviour*' they adopt (see below).

What is ill health? Disease, illness and sickness

In everyday life we tend to use these terms almost interchangeably, but it is useful to distinguish them for analytical purposes to help clarify different dimensions of suffering in the biopsychosocial model. Thus *disease* can be defined as organic pathology or abnormality (though the extent to which an abnormality can or should be classified as a disease is a matter for debate in medicine and in society in general). *Illness* is the subjective experience of, and meaning attributed to, ill health by the patient and those around him or her. Disease

is often described as the doctor's perspective, illness as the patient's perspective. *Sickness* is the social, external and public recognition of ill health, and is dependent on a number of factors, not least, often, having a disease. A sick person occupies a social role (the 'sick role'), which is dependent on society for its recognition and maintenance (see Chapter 6). We could say that disease resides in the organism, illness resides in the person and sickness resides in society.

What is a disease?

In the biomedical model, a disease is the product of a causative agent (a pathogen) on a susceptible organism, and its biological consequences. The pathogen can be genetic, developmental, environmental, or a combination of all three. Identification of the disease (diagnosis) leads to a specific treatment and cure.

What is an illness?

An illness is the subjective, psychological experience of ill health. The illness may have a biological basis, but this is not essential. The experience of illness is generally one of a move from independence to dependence and is strongly influenced by social and economic factors. For example, depression in the UK is strongly linked to gender and class, with women demonstrating a 2:1 rate for depression. Working-class women are particularly at risk compared to their middle-class counterparts, because they are more likely to experience the vulnerabilities associated with depression (e.g. unemployment) and to experience a provoking agent (e.g. a serious life event or major difficulty).

What is a sickness?

Sickness is the social experience of ill health – what happens when a disease or illness is acknowledged and dealt with in the public sphere. Sickness can be thought of as all those aspects of disease or illness which make them more than a purely biological or psychological reality. For example, many diseases and/or illnesses raise economic and political or legal issues (the issuance of sick notes, for example). It is also the case that particular diseases occupy a certain position in the collective consciousness or imagination of the community.

To help clarify the above definitions, it may be possible to imagine examples where a disease is not associated with any illness or sickness, and of an illness which is neither a disease nor sickness. Even where a disease or illness is lacking there can still be sickness, socially defined. Such forms of sickness may not be regarded as medically signifi-

cant, but they often contribute to more biological or psychological forms of ill health, or have physiological or psychological consequences. (See Figure 2.2.)

Examples of disease without illness or sickness ('labelling')

Hypertension
HIV-positive status
A suspect cervical smear

Examples of illness without disease or sickness

Hypochondria
Malingering

Examples of sickness without disease or illness

Racism
Prejudice
Violence

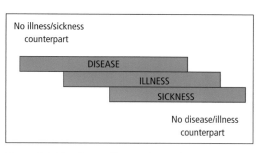

Figure 2.2 The disease/illness/sickness distinction.

Case study: Disease, illness and sickness

Lorna, aged 45, was recalled to her GP because the results of her cervical smear indicated she might have a malignancy. She had been feeling fine and had been invited for a smear as all women should be, once every four years, as part of a routine screening programme.

Beatrice, an elderly, recently widowed lady, attended her GP again because she continued to be anxious about her lower intestine. She was experiencing acute pain and discomfort in her lower bowel and was convinced she had something wrong, even though earlier investigations by colonoscopy and barium meal had both indicated nothing suspicious. Her GP could only assume there was nothing wrong and that Beatrice was a hypochondriac.

Stan, a 50-year-old father of four, visited his GP for a sick note. He needed it, he thought, to be put on incapacity benefit for his bad back. His discussion with the doctor led into talking about conditions on his housing estate. This estate, built in the 1960s by the local council, was known locally as 'the reservation'. Recently, some 'problem families' had moved in and had made conditions much less tolerable. Now there were muggings, tyre slashing, joy-riding and racist taunts directed at Stan and his family – there were many ways in which life on the estate had got worse in recent years.

Identify which of these cases is an example that is predominantly concerned with disease, which is predominantly concerned with illness and which is predominantly concerned with sickness.

Explanations of ill health

Notions of disease causality are another important factor explaining people's health-seeking behaviour. What explanations for suffering do people hold? These can be divided into four categories: individual, environmental/natural, social and supernatural.

Explanations of ill health

Individual causes, e.g.
  sin/breach of taboos
  soul theft
  immune system weakness
Natural causes, e.g.
  germs
  humoral imbalance
  hot/cold imbalance
  fate/bad luck
Social causes, e.g.
  sorcery, witchcraft, the evil eye
Supernatural causes, e.g.
  punishment from God/spirit/ancestor

Not all these explanations would be acceptable in a biomedical approach to ill health. In order to understand them, we need to know more about the worldview of particular cultures and the individuals within them. Soul theft, for example, is regarded as a serious condition in certain parts of the world, caused by the soul wandering at night in dreams. It is dangerous to wake someone in the middle of a dream in case the soul fails to return to the body it has left. Loss of the soul leads to serious illness and death, unless special rituals are conducted to retrieve it.

Not all cultures differentiate between the causes of ill health and the causes of other kinds of misfortune. Breaking taboos can be held responsible not only for certain types of illness, but also for crop failure. Sin may also be regarded as causing ill health, either through the dangers inherent in the sinful behaviour itself or through the risks it poses of divine punishment.

Obviously, what is perceived as causing an illness is going to affect how it is treated, and sometimes multiple theories can be held. For example, it may be accepted that germs have caused an illness, but God's punishment is seen as the ultimate cause. Hence two forms of treatment may be sought, sometimes simultaneously.

Labelling and stigma

Labelling is the social significance attributed to an act linked to an individual or a group, such as the attachment of a medical diagnosis to someone. Labelling can be positive, but is usually negative. Often, a person's outlook and behaviour can be changed dramatically due to the label that has been applied. For example, a middle-aged woman experiencing the early symptoms of angina may regard them as essentially harmless. A diagnosis of coronary heart disease (CHD) not only presents various treatment options, but also what can be a devastating future for the woman who is now a patient. She is frightened; she may stop smoking, give up drinking and try a low-cholesterol diet. She may become extremely concerned about over-exertion in case it places undue stress on her heart. Her husband is also worried about her over-exerting herself and discourages her from doing the gardening she used to enjoy. She is unable to get additional life insurance (assuming she has some in the first place) because of prohibitively high premiums. In short, her life has been transformed.

The results of labelling are particularly marked in circumstances where either the patient previously regarded the symptoms as harmless or felt perfectly healthy.

HIV-positive status can have a similarly transforming effect on a people's lives, making them depressed, introspective and perhaps prompting major changes in their sexual activity. An HIV-positive person has to decide to whom to disclose the HIV status to, knowing that disclosure may fundamentally change the attitude of the person told to the person making the disclosure. As with CHD, a diagnosis of HIV affects an individual's ability to obtain life insurance, as well as employment prospects.

A label that invokes a negative social reaction results in 'stigma'. Stigma is a mark of social disgrace. It varies across time and place (e.g. in attitudes to births out of wedlock, or to homosexuality) (see Table 2.2; see also Chapter 12).

Table 2.2 The anatomy of stigma.

Type of stigma	Examples
Discreditable stigma – keeping potentially stigmatizing conditions hidden from all but one's closest intimates.	• That someone is HIV-positive. • Someone who has had a mastectomy or an ileostomy never going to a swimming pool or getting undressed in the presence of strangers.
Managing the control of information about a potentially stigmatizing condition can be very stressful	
Discrediting stigma – when a potentially stigmatizing condition cannot be hidden	• Someone with acne. • Someone with an amputation, who uses a wheelchair, or who has lost a sensory organ.
Such a person must deal with the assumptions and judgements of others about their situation. A common complaint of someone with a stigmatized condition is that people respond to them on the basis of their visible difference rather than to them as a person	
Felt stigma – the fear an individual or group may have that they and their condition will be negatively viewed.	• Someone with a sexually transmitted infection attending a GUM clinic for the first time.
This is only internally experienced	
Enacted stigma – the actual, first-hand experience of stigma	• Someone with schizophrenia being ordered off a bus.
Cultural stereotyping – the result of collective attitudes that groups hold towards a stigmatized condition Cultural stereotyping may lead to prejudice, discrimination and disadvantage for the person with the condition	• Substance abusers hiding their habit from an employer.
Self-fulfilling prophecy – belief that cultural stereotypes will mean the person will be devalued and discriminated against. Such assumptions result in coping strategies being adopted such as secrecy and social withdrawal. These have consequences for quality of life and reinforce the feeling of stigma	• People with anorexia nervosa attempting to conceal their condition.
Secondary deviation – further behaviour change in the individual suffering from the stigmatized condition as a result of either felt or enacted stigma.	• Knowledge that others consider them incapable, for example, may lead to those with disabilities adopting a position of 'learned helplessness' about their condition.
Courtesy stigma – stigma that is not experienced directly. Sometimes a carer may feel ashamed of or embarrassed by the person with a stigmatized condition they are somehow responsible for	• Parents taking their child who has autism to a restaurant. • The spouse or partner of someone with Alzheimer's disease being embarrassed about them shouting.

The process of stigmatization

1 People differentiate and label differences that are considered socially important.

2 People thus labelled are placed in distinct categories (e.g. 'fat', 'disabled', 'epileptic', 'schizophrenic') that separate them from 'normal' people.

3 Cultural beliefs link these differences to other attributes, many of them reliant on negative stereotypes (e.g. people with mental illness are a danger to others).

4 People who are labelled are therefore devalued, experiencing loss of status and discrimination (e.g. unequal health care and socio–economic disadvantage).

5 This process is dependent on and perpetuated by the social, economic and political power of those doing the labelling, separating, stereotyping and discriminating.

Table 2.3 Changing the label: an attempt to deal with stigma.

Old, discredited label	New, correct label
Madness	Mental illness
Spasticity	Cerebral palsy
Mongolism	Down syndrome
Leprosy	Hansen's disease

Some of the types of stigma in Table 2.2 overlap as there are no hard-and-fast rules about what stigma is. Because of the stigma associated with particular conditions, sometimes attempts have been made to overcome it by changing the name of the condition (Table 2.3).

In addition to renaming diseases it is also good practice, for example, not to refer to 'the paraplegic' or 'the schizophrenic' but to the person (or people) with paraplegia/schizophrenia. The good doctor considers the effects of labelling on the patient in every case.

The body

People's ideas about the body can have significant health implications. Ideas about size, shape, adornment, structure and functioning all affect people's health and illness behaviour. In the UK, the ideas people have are increasingly influenced by medical science. The body is not only a physical object – or if it is a physical object it is one that is disagreed about and a site where many of the tensions of modern society are displayed. It is a place where notions of beauty, ideal body shape and what is fashionable manifest themselves through diet, clothing, tattooing, piercing, plastic surgery and circumcision. Our conceptions about the body often derive from technological innovations that then become the basis of metaphorical descriptions – plumbing, for example, or computers. The machine metaphor that characterizes western biomedicine resonates strongly in the popular sector. For example, a familiar brand of car maintenance manual has recently started producing popular books in the same style such as 'The Man Manual' and 'The Woman Manual' in a clever play on this tendency.

'Body language', the gestures people use and the postures they adopt, is an important form of non-verbal communication and one that we use constantly (and relatively unconsciously) to assess things about a person's position in society: age, gender, social status, occupation and group membership, for example. As well as its more utilitarian function of protecting the body from the environment, clothing signals much the same sorts of things. These messages and their interpretation differ between cultures and between different groups and individuals within cultures. Sometimes clothing can have health consequences: corsetry and high-heeled shoes are examples of clothing designed to accentuate desirable features in women that have health implications.

Artificial changes in the shape, size and body surface (skin) are widely made throughout the world, and may also serve a communicative function. Sometimes the boundary between self-expression and self-mutilation may be difficult to draw.

Examples of artificial changes in the body common in the UK

- Tanning using UV sunbeds
- Ear piercing
- Nose piercing
- Other body piercings – tongue, lip, eyebrow, nipple, genitalia
- Male circumcision
- Tattooing
- Cosmetic dentistry
- Plastic surgery

In addition there are other forms of body mutilation that may be seen among migrants to the UK. Among these is female circumcision, which is particularly prevalent in parts of sub-Sahara Africa, parts of the Arab world, Malaysia and Indonesia. It is estimated that 80 million women and girls alive today have undergone circumcision, involving the removal of all or part of the external genitalia. This compares with male circumcision, which it is estimated has been experienced by 750 million boys and men worldwide and is a religious requirement of Judaism and Islam. In the United States, male circumcision is routinely practised on infants in the majority of cases, generally in medical settings, despite the fact that medical opinion is divided as to whether there is any health-related value to it (or what the risks might be). For this reason, medical circumcision has been described as 'an operation in search of a disease'. It is a prime example of the power of society in shaping medical practice.

Body structure and function

Most members of the lay public have never been involved in an anatomical dissection; nor are they expert in their comprehension of human physiology. They thus base much of their knowledge of body structure and function on common-sense notions picked up at different stages of the life course, books and the media. Such knowledge affects their perceptions of the body and its malfunctions, how they present to the doctor, and their responses to medical treatment. Studies of lay perceptions of internal anatomy have found major differences between these and the perceptions of doctors. For example, nearly 60% of participants in a British study conducted in the late 1960s thought that the stomach was positioned in the area from just under the breast to the groin (a conception that is also common in Jamaica). 'Stomach pain' may thus refer to pain in a large part of the abdominal cavity and should be interpreted by the doctor with caution.

Lay theories of body function can be loosely grouped around those concerning the need for *balance* and those concerning the need for *flow*. Just as lay beliefs about body structure can have clinical significance, so do lay beliefs about body function. These beliefs are changing, partly through the influence of biomedical knowledge and practice and partly because of changing technologies which give people different models and metaphors to use in thinking about their bodies. With industrialization, the body came to be seen more like a factory with inputs (e.g. food) and outputs (e.g. waste products). Plumbing metaphors have also become popular (e.g. likening one's urinary tract to 'waterworks') and in recent years the brain has come to be thought of less like a telephone exchange and more like a computer.

Balance and imbalance in body function

The need for balance within the body is a belief shared by many expressions in biomedical practice such as hormone imbalances, vitamin deficiencies and bacterial overload. As in lay beliefs, such balance is regarded as depending on external influences such as diet or the environment, or on internal workings such as state of mind. One of the most widespread theories of balance which persists in lay beliefs (and to a certain extent in biomedical beliefs) worldwide is the *humoral* system. This sees the body as made up of four humours – blood, phlegm, yellow bile and black bile. Balancing the humours is the basis of good health and is achieved through managing the influences of diet, the seasons, activities, sex, age and personal relationships. The humoral system has its roots in ancient Chinese and Indian medicine, but was elaborated by Hippocrates, the father of western medicine (see Chapter 4).

Other health systems are based on the principle of '*hot/cold*' balance. These terms do not necessarily correspond to 'hot' and 'cold' as we use them in English to denote temperature, but more to a symbolic power contained in many natural substances, mental states, illnesses and supernatural forces. Certain 'hot' illnesses are perceived as resulting from over-exposure to the sun, fire, hot food or drinks. Pregnancy and menstruation in many Latin American and Caribbean countries are regarded as 'hot' states and therefore vulnerable to the influence of 'cold' substances such as foods regarded as 'cold'. In biomedical terms, some of these 'cold' fruit and vegetables would be beneficial to women's health. Similar problems occur in parts of Pakistan where infant diarrhoea is regarded as a 'cold' disease and one in which giving fluids to replace the water lost in the stools is seen as simply adding to the problem. Such beliefs can have fatal consequences for the vulnerable infant.

English folk beliefs about 'colds' and 'chills' are also influenced by humoral thinking: in both cases the cold, damp climate has penetrated the body and has to be counteracted by warming drinks, warm foods and rest in a warm place. GPs in many cases share these beliefs with their patients.

Ideas of flow in body function

Just as 'balance' is regarded as important to health, so for many people 'flow' is important in maintaining good respiratory, cardiovascular, intestinal and genitourinary health. Numerous products flow – blood, air, food, faeces, urine, menstrual blood – and disease is caused by blockage of this flow in some way. In the UK, for example, constipation is a common complaint. Among the older generation in particular, retained faeces are believed to release toxins and impurities into the blood, which affect both complexion and overall health.

Case study: The 'three piece suite'

Alan is visiting his GP:
GP: What seems to be the problem?
Alan: It's a bit difficult to explain, really. You see, it's the three piece suite.
GP [completely baffled]: The three piece suite? What's wrong with it?
Alan: It's the colour – it's wrong.
GP [uncertain why a patient should be bringing his furniture problems to the surgery]: Your three piece suite is the wrong colour? How can I help you with that?
Alan: By sorting it out for me, of course!
GP [starting to feel a bit rattled]: I don't understand – you want me to deal with your furniture problem?
Alan [laughing]: Not me furniture, no. Y'know, me 'meat and two veg' – there's a rash you see!

The confusion in the above case study is due to the embarrassment Alan feels about talking about his genitalia with a stranger. Other parts of the body may elicit similar feelings of shame and embarrassment – for example, the rectum and anus (see Case Study in Chapter 8).

Summary

Models of health and ill health have clinical relevance in the following ways:

- Health models are culturally derived and are associated with particular social categories such as age, class and gender, affecting people's patterns of 'health-seeking behaviour'.

• Different health models and explanations of ill health affect the expectations patients have of medical personnel and the treatment options they follow.

• The social labelling of particular illnesses may lead to stigmatization of the sufferer. This can be of several different types.

• People's ideas about the body may have significant clinical and behavioural implications.

• Understanding patients' ideas, concerns and expectations about health and ill health and the body are important in providing high quality care – patient-centred medicine.

Further reading

Aggleton, P. (1990) *Health*. London: Routledge.

Blaxter, M. (1990) *Health and Lifestyles*. London: Tavistock.

Blaxter, M. (2004) *Health*. Cambridge: Polity Press.

Helman, C. (2007) *Culture, Health and Illness* (5th edn.). London: Hodder Arnold. Chapter 2: The body: cultural definitions of anatomy and physiology.

Scambler, G. (2003) Deviance, sick role and stigma. In G. Scambler (ed.) *Sociology as Applied to Medicine*. London: Saunders.

Seedhouse, D. (1986). *Health: the Foundations for Achievement*. Chichester: Wiley

Weston, W. W. and Brown, J. B. (1995) Overview of the patient-centred clinical method. In M. Stewart et al. *Patient-Centred Medicine: Transforming the Clinical Method*. Thousand Oaks, CA: Sage.

Chapter 3

Health and health care in the popular sector

Introduction

The popular sector and what happens in it are the major determining influence on people's health and the therapeutic strategies that are employed to deal with ill health. The popular sector is the domain of health care that takes place without reference to a 'folk' or 'professional' healer. A defining feature of health care in the popular sector is that it is unpaid. The 2001 Census indicated that one in ten UK adults is a carer, defined as 'someone who, without payment, provides help and support to a relative, friend, child or neighbour who could not manage without their help'. Estimates vary, but it is likely that the cost of this care, if left to the state, would be in the region of £57 billion a year. While many of the carers are elderly, the 2001 Census identified 13,000 young people aged under 18 years who were spending more than 50 hours a week caring for someone else. Their needs are also important as inevitably their education and social life are curtailed by such a commitment.

The family is the arena for much of this caring activity, as well as being a major determinant of the health or ill health of its members in the first place. Moving outwards from 'the family', there is

increasing recognition of the role played by wider social networks and 'social capital' as determinants of health, ill health and health care. There is a significant 'illness iceberg' of symptoms that are not brought to the attention of medical practitioners, and understanding the reasons for people's decisions to consult a GP, and the kinds of treatment they expect and use, are vital for effective, patient-centred care.

> **This chapter covers the following topics**
>
> Experience of illness in the popular sector
> Social organization of the popular sector
> Health care options in the popular sector
> Health-seeking behaviour

Experience of illness in the popular sector

In any two-week period, 75% of the UK population will experience one or more symptoms of ill health. Yet the proportion of people with symptoms who will consult their GP or other health professional about them is minimal. There is an 'illness iceberg' of symptoms about which people do nothing, self-medicate or consult an alternative or complementary practitioner (Figure 3.1).

One study conducted in 1980 asked 79 women aged 16–44 years living on a London housing estate to keep diaries for six weeks in which they

Lecture Notes: *The Social Basis of Medicine*, 1st edition. By Andrew Russell. Published 2009 by Blackwell Publishing. ISBN: 978-1-4051-3912-0

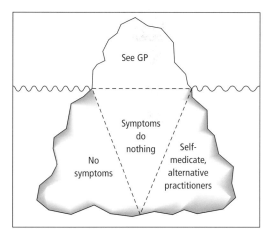

Figure 3.1 The illness iceberg.

The differences, shown in Table 3.1, are important because if there was any significant change in consultation patterns with regard to any of these symptoms, the primary care services would be swamped. While in this case the symptoms may be regarded as mild and not indicative of disease requiring medical treatment, a much larger study of 3160 adults attending a mobile health clinic found that 57% had health problems that were referred to their GP for further tests and possible treatment. More than one third of these problems had not previously been reported to the GP, and 22% (264 people) were judged serious enough to warrant a hospital referral. There is therefore an unmet need from people who are sustaining avoidable pain, discomfort and handicap due to symptoms which are treatable. On the other hand, GPs complain of a widespread tendency for people to consult for trivial or inappropriate reasons. Understanding the causes of 'health-seeking behaviour', then, has important implications for medical practice.

recorded any symptoms and consultations. During this time, the women recorded 863 symptoms, of which 49 prompted a consultation with a doctor. The ratio of consultation to symptom episodes varied markedly, reflecting different beliefs and experiences of particular symptoms.

Table 3.1 Symptom episodes and medical consultations recorded in London women's health diaries (Source: Scambler et al. 1981, Royal College of General Practitioners).

Main types of symptoms recorded	No. of symptom episodes	No. of occasions leading to consultation	Ratio of medical consultation: symptom episodes
Headache	180	3	1:60
Changes in energy, tiredness	109	0	–
Nerves, depression, irritability	74	1	1:74
Aches or pains in joints, muscles, legs or arms	71	4	1:18
Women's complaints (e.g. period pain)	69	7	1:10
Stomach aches or pains	45	4	1:11
Backache	38	1	1:38
Cold, 'flu, runny nose	37	3	1:12
Sore throat	36	4	1:9
Sleeplessness	31	1	1:31
Others	173	21	1:8
Totals	**863**	**49**	**1:18**

Social organization in the popular sector

The *family* is a key element of health care in this sector. One definition of the family is 'a married or cohabiting couple on their own or with their never married children who have no children of their own or lone parents and similar such children'. Sometimes such a family is 'extended' by the addition of relatives from other generations or branches of the family tree (e.g. aunts and uncles). While people may stereotypically consider a 'nuclear' family of a married couple and their average 1.8 dependent children as the 'typical' household type in the UK, the 2001 Census showed that only 18% of households fit this pattern (a further 3% were made up of cohabiting couples with dependent children). Seven per cent of households were made up of a lone parent with dependent children; 35% of households were of a married or cohabiting couple without children or with non-dependent children (2% of households were lone parents without dependent children); and 31% of households were made up of one person only, of whom nearly half were one pensioner-only households, and of these three-quarters (2.34 million) were women living alone.

These figures are the result of changes which have been taking place in the UK over the past 100 years (Table 3.2).

Families are important also for the genetic, environmental and demographic predispositions they bring to bear on individual members. Shopping, cooking, cleaning and washing are tasks that may be taken for granted, but they have profound implications for maintaining health. Families act not only as a source of direct care but also as mediators between the patient and his or her dealings with the folk and professional sectors (see Chapters 5 and 4 respectively), particularly if the problem is serious. The entire range of people involved in the patient's care is known collectively as his or her *therapy managing group*, and such groups are a universal phenomenon. When therapy managing groups are necessary, those without family members living nearby are at a disadvantage unless mechanisms are in place to ensure alternative forms of support are available. The increasing mobility of families means that the elderly may be unsupported and their relatives face particular problems attempting

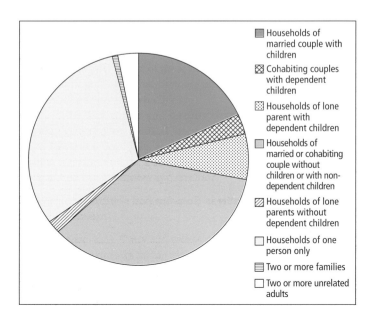

- Households of married couple with children
- Cohabiting couples with dependent children
- Households of lone parent with dependent children
- Households of married or cohabiting couple without children or with non-dependent children
- Households of lone parents without dependent children
- Households of one person only
- Two or more families
- Two or more unrelated adults

Figure 3.2 Household structure in the UK, 2001 (Source: Living in Britain 2001, National Statistics: www.statistics.gov.uk)

Table 3.2 Historical changes in UK families.

Increases in	Decreases in
Average age at first marriage	Percentage living in 'nuclear' families of married couple and dependent children
Cohabitation	Average completed family size
Remarriage	Marriages per year
Average age of primiparous (first-time) mother	Average age of mother at birth of final child
Births outside marriage	
Single-parent families	
Reconstituted families	

to care 'at a distance'. Other health results of the changes in family life over the past 100 years include the increased risk of poverty, child care burdens, stress and nutritional problems often faced by single-parent families, and the stress, emotional disruption to children, adult depression and poorer nutrition associated with relationship breakdown. However, it is important to avoid stereotyping different types of families or making assumptions about families that are different in structure from one's own. Many families exhibit 'positive deviance', i.e. characteristics that 'buck the trend' or the patterns outlined above. Reconstituted families can be very warm and supportive places for children and adults:

the stereotype of the wicked stepmother or stepfather in children's literature is just that – a stereotype!

Illness also impacts on the family. Women – wives, mothers and daughters – provide the bulk of health care in the popular sector and hence bear a particular burden in times of ill health. Roles and relationships can be transformed by the biographical disruption brought by a longstanding chronic illness. Illness and disability in a child may affect well siblings, who may feel or actually be neglected because of the attention that is paid to the child with problems.

Families can also negatively affect the health of members.

Case study: The effect of childhood asthma on families

One in eight children has asthma, a six-fold increase over the past 25 years. A study conducted in the late 1980s indicated how the health status of one family member with asthma can seriously affect the emotional and material well-being of all other members. Here are some of the examples the study found:
- Parents taking less well-paid jobs nearer home to be closer to children.
- Emergency care meant time off work and hence loss of earnings.
- One-off costs (such as new bedding) and regular costs (such as hospital visits) were a financial drain.
- Asthma attacks and the disrupted sleep for all family members that ensue lead to tiredness, irritability and lack of concentration.

Case study: Domestic violence as a 'family affair'

It is estimated that one in four women will experience domestic violence at some point in their lives. Domestic violence features in at least 25% of all divorces in England and Wales, and every year 63,000 women and children spend at least one night in a refuge escaping a violent husband/partner and father. Approximately one women every three days dies in the UK as a result of domestic violence. It is found in all social classes and ethnic groups, yet is often 'hidden' from professional help. The victims of domestic violence are frequently too afraid to come forward, or else

(continued on p. 28)

(continued)

attribute injuries to another source (e.g. 'I walked into a door'). Health professionals have a tendency not to ask the obvious question: 'Have you been a victim of domestic violence?'

In addition to the physical and psychological scars borne by the direct victim of the abuse, those who have witnessed it, such as their children, may present with a variety of health problems, including physical assaults, anxiety, depression and eating disorders. While domestic violence is primarily experienced by women, men are the victims in up to 10% of cases. Children also experience high levels of physical assaults and emotional abuse.

The elderly are also subject to psychological and physical abuse perpetrated by family members or those paid to look after them. One survey suggested that one in three old people suffer some kind of psychological abuse, and 20% are physically abused, financially exploited or otherwise subject to 'undue influence' from people who do not necessarily have the older person's best interest at heart. Sometimes the abusers are family members.

Except where families are estranged or where members live apart with little contact, families form an important part of the *social network* of an individual. A social network is a map of the relationships among people indicating the ways in which they are connected. Like the family, the social network a person is in can have a profound influence on their health and the sort of health-seeking behaviour they adopt. Networks can be analysed according to the number and frequency of contacts as well as the density of the network of which the person is a part (i.e. the number of people a person knows). However, as well as these more quantitative measures it is important to take into account the type and quality of contact involved.

Case study: Susie's social networks

Figure 3.3 shows three 'contact groups' – Susie's family, where the network is densest, and two groups of (we presume) friends. The two groups of friends are separate, as are the friends and her family. We cannot tell from the figure the frequency of contacts with people in each group or what the nature of that contact is (e.g. face-to-face, phone calls, text messaging).

Susie was a heroin user, and the figure was drawn by an addictions nurse in conversation with Susie as a means of clarifying the networks that Susie had. Susie's friends in the lower right part of the figure were her 'heroin pals'. However, the nurse could ascertain that Susie had good potential support from other friends who did not use heroin and from her family.

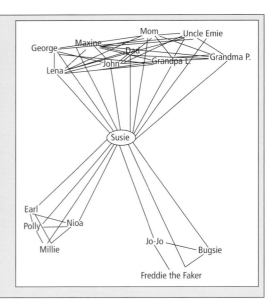

Figure 3.3 Contact groups for Susie.

Well-functioning families are an important source of support for an individual in times of ill health, but dysfunctional families can negatively affect the health of their members; so can the social networks an individual is embedded in. Here the quality of those networks is an important source of health or cause of ill health. The support provided by social networks can act as a buffer against the effects of stress and be a source of esteem and well-being irrespective of stress. On the other hand, social ties can be harmful. It is unlikely that Susie's health benefited greatly from her association with her 'heroin pals'; similarly, being a member of a criminal gang is unlikely to be a health-promoting experience. There are many ways in which social relationships can encourage unhealthy behaviour.

Health care options in the popular sector

> **Options available to people in the popular sector**
>
> - Lay referral networks
> - Self-treatment or self-medication
> - Self-help groups

Lay referral networks

Unless they live alone and are isolated from other people, most people will discuss their symptoms with another person. The social networks through which individuals pass before seeking professional advice are known as lay referral networks. They consist of any advice or treatment given by relatives, friends, neighbours or colleagues. Sometimes particular people in the community will figure highly in such a network, for example those with experience of a specific illness, those with experience raising children or those who are or have been health professionals. The lay referral system used will affect whether professional care is sought and, if it is, the type of care sought. In the London study outlined above, there were 11 lay consultations for every medical one.

The outcome of lay referral will largely depend on the beliefs, attitudes, resources and access to formal health care of the individual with symptoms and the other network members. If the network has beliefs and circumstances that are incongruent with those of doctors, then uptake of medical services may be relatively low. For example, if the symptom does not deviate from culturally defined 'normality' (e.g. persistent cough among a family of smokers; constant tiredness among new parents), then the symptom is unlikely to be validated to encourage attendance at a medical service. The kind of network

consulted also appears to be important; in the London study kinship networks appeared to be more likely to encourage consultations than friendship networks.

Self-treatment or self-medication

Self-treatment, specifically self-medication, forms a major part of health care in the popular sector. It includes home remedies and over-the-counter (OTC) medications. A study in 1972 found lower consultation rates among people who reported self-medication and that in a two-week period two-thirds of a sample population of adults had taken at least one non-prescribed medication, exceeding prescribed medication by a ratio of 2:1. Most of these non-prescribed medications had been recommended by members of a lay referral network; only 10% had been suggested by a doctor. Adults tend to use self-medication as a substitute for a GP consultation. In some cases what they use is not medically approved: for example, in 2006 the Mental Health Foundation published figures claiming that 12 million adults in the UK use alcohol as a form of 'self-medication' for stress, anxiety and depression.

Children are other primary users of non-prescribed medicines since they are largely dependent on their parent or other carer for access to medication. For them, self- or parent-medication seems to be used more as an adjunct to medical consultation. One study of mothers with young children found that self-care was the principal way in which children's symptoms were dealt with. In 65% of cases where some kind of change was noticed that might indicate illness, mothers took action, although in only 10% cases did this involve making contact with a health professional. By 'catching illness early', mothers saw themselves as reducing the likelihood of having to go to their GP for a prescribed medicine. They were reluctant to bother the doctor with trivial symptoms and knew from their own experience that many symptoms are self-limiting. Some of the actions they took might have been previously recommended by doctors or health professionals. The pharmacist was an important part of the lay

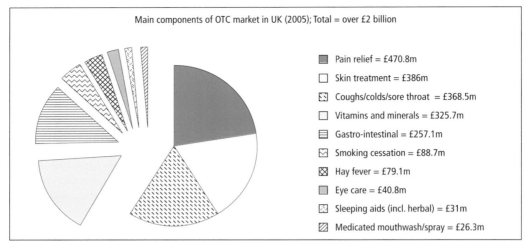

Figure 3.4 The over-the-counter market in the UK, 2005 (Source: www.pagb.org.uk).

referral system, a source in particular of analgesics and cough medicines.

Drug deregulation has led to an increase in the number of OTC medicines being made available. One of the latest of these is statin self-medication to reduce blood cholesterol, which became available OTC in 2004. Some welcome the greater autonomy and consumer choice permitted with regard to medicine taking (although some of the more expensive drugs would be free of charge for the majority of the population who are exempt from the prescription charge). Some GPs advise their prescription-paying patients to buy an OTC drug rather than obtain it on prescription as it is cheaper that way (e.g. hydrocortisone cream). However, the efficacy of some traditional medications, such as expectorant for cough, is not well proven, and the opportunity for misuse of pharmaceutical products of all sorts is ever present. The role of the community pharmacist is being developed in an effort to bridge the gap between the popular and professional sectors. The pharmacist may give health advice, although in many cases consumers use the pharmacy (or supermarket) to purchase the products they have used before for similar symptoms. Whether as an adjunct or alternative to going to the doctor, pharmacists seem destined to fulfil an increasingly important role in self-care (see Figure 3.4).

Self-help groups

Self-help health groups are designed to help those with a condition either through services for individual sufferers and their carers or by lobbying for changes in attitudes or health care provision at the local, regional and national levels. They have grown rapidly in recent years, so that in the UK a self-help group exists for just about every long-term health condition, whether defined as an illness or other 'deviation from the norm'. This is partly because of the increasing number of conditions for which existing services seem inadequate and partly because of the general tendency for people to want to take more control and responsibility for the management of their condition, and for the government to encourage this to happen. As with activities in other parts of the popular sector, it is members' experience rather than their education that is important, especially direct or indirect experience of a particular misfortune. The work of such groups can provide an alternative or be an adjunct to formal medical care.

Examples of national self-help groups (with website addresses)

Action on Elder Abuse (www.elderabuse.org.uk)
Alcoholics Anonymous (www.alcoholics-anonymous.org.uk)

Arthritis Care (www.arthritiscare.org.uk)

Child Bereavement Trust (www.childbereavement.org.uk)

Colostomy Association (www.colostomyassociation.org.uk)

CRUSE Bereavement Care (www.crusebereavementcare.org.uk)

Cystic Fibrosis Trust (www.cftrust.org.uk)

Diabetes UK (www.diabetes.org.uk)

Down's Syndrome Support Group (www.dsa-uk.com)

Eating Disorders Association (www.edauk.com)

Gamblers Anonymous (www.gamblersanonymous.org.uk)

Gingerbread (www.gingerbread.org.uk)

ME Association (www.meassociation.org.uk)

MESMAC (www.mesmac.co.uk)

MIND (www.mind.org.uk)

Multiple Sclerosis Society (www.mssociety.org.uk)

Narcotics Anonymous (www.ukna.org)

National Association for People Abused in Childhood (www.napac.org.uk)

National Federation of Solo Clubs (myweb.tiscali.co.uk/solofederation)

Overeaters Anonymous (www.oagb.org.uk)

Parkinson's Disease Society (www.parkinsons.org.uk)

Psoriasis Association (www.psoriasis-association.org.uk)

Rethink (previously the 'National Schizophrenia Fellowship') (www.rethink.org)

Riding for the Disabled Association (www.riding-for-disabled.org.uk)

University of the Third Age (www.u3a.org.uk)

Women's Aid and Refuge (www.womensaid.org.uk)

The purposes for which self-help groups are formed span many types of physical illnesses and disability and illnesses which are more contested (such as the ME [Myalgic Encephalopathy] Association), or addictions (Alcoholics Anonymous; Gamblers Anonymous; Overeaters Anonymous) and traumatic life events (The Child Bereavement Trust; CRUSE Bereavement Care). Some groups (such as Rethink) have traditionally worked more with carers, while others (such as MIND) work on a more personal, social and political level. The Psoriasis Association is an example of a group that spans the popular and professional sector, since its membership includes sufferers and their relatives, doctors, nurses, and cosmetic and pharmaceutical companies. Other groups are more anti-professional in their stance and hostile to orthodox medicine. People tend to seek out groups that support their personal philosophy, which may differ from current professional thinking. Where opinions differ within or between groups, tensions and even hostility may arise.

Some groups are not specifically concerned with 'health' *per se* but cover an array of social problems such as those faced by one-parent families (Gingerbread) or loneliness (The National Federation of Solo Clubs and even an organization such as the University of the Third Age). MESMAC (Men who have Sex with Men Action in the Community) has social groups throughout the north of England. These also provide advice and information on safe sex, counselling for men who have been the victims of partner abuse, and advice and support for those living with HIV (organizations, such as the various branches of Body Positive, are more specifically geared for those with HIV). There are many organizations, not listed above, that cater for the specific needs of ethnic minority groups, women and children.

The functions that these groups perform also overlap and groups may operate in a number of different ways. For particularly stigmatized or disadvantaged people, the group may provide the main source of social contact, friendship and *support*. Those who have learned to live with their condition may act as powerful *role models* in some cases, and in others can provide advice on *coping strategies* that is often better than that offered by most health professionals. Many groups provide important *information and advice* about the condition. *Mutual aid* and *empowerment* are two other ways in which self-help groups provide support for those who need it.

The development of community care has pushed some groups that were previously support and advice organizations into being service providers. Organizations have been successful in obtaining grants that enable them to provide services directly to client groups rather than just members so that the boundary between self-help groups and voluntary organizations has become increasingly fuzzy. There are advantages and disadvantages to these changes. Services provided by self-help organizations tend to be more closely tailored to users' needs and those involved can have more of a say in the running of the services. On the other hand, self-help projects usually suffer from short-term funding and insecurity and are too often expected to plug gaps in service provision where more money would otherwise be required to provide adequate resources to statutory and professional organizations. Groups lose their mutual aid focus, and staff can be brought in to run the organization and its services who do not have the same ethos or concern for the centrality of the user's experience. As they become more dependent on money from donors who can then 'call the shots', in their move to fund services some of the more dynamic social and political activism of such groups may be lost.

While most self-help groups provide the opportunity for face-to-face or at least phone contact, nowadays they almost always provide some kind of website to advertise and support their work. Other groups are now starting up solely on the internet. The internet can offer support outside one's immediate area, as well as anonymity where the individual is experiencing stigmatization. In some cases people with a particular condition may find it more stigmatizing to socialize with other sufferers than with 'normal' friends and relatives. For those with a long-term degenerative condition such as multiple sclerosis, it can be depressing to meet people who are 'further down the line' of deterioration than they are. The internet is also an important source of help for those with mobility

problems or who live in remote communities. On the other hand, the internet can promote non-standard approaches to conditions that may be of questionable benefit. For example, there are many sites promoting anorexia nervosa as a lifestyle choice rather than an illness and offering advice on to how become anorexic.

Points of view

Self-help groups
- Complementary or subversive?
- A poor substitute for people starved of real services?
- A basic component of primary health care?
- Is home the most dangerous place in modern society?

Health-seeking behaviour

Health-seeking behaviour may be defined as the ways in which individuals, families, communities and other groups seek to maintain and improve health (health-seeking behaviour), and deal with ill-health (illness behaviour). This section considers the ways in which the popular sector influences people's decision-making with regard to accessing health care.

Triggers to consult

The motivating factor in the decision to consult a GP for a particular symptom or symptoms is known as the 'trigger to consult'. Triggers can be classified as 'cultural', 'social' or 'practical'.

Types of triggers to consult

Cultural
- Fear that symptoms may indicate something more sinister (derives from beliefs about symptoms and causes).
- Knowledge of what is available and its suitability for the symptoms identified.
- Experience, direct as patient or indirect as carer or by carer(s), that influences perceptions about likely efficacy of treatment (i.e. cure or amelioration of symptoms).
- The compatibility of illness recognition between the patient, their family and other carers, and the healer involved.

Social
- The occurrence of an interpersonal crisis (e.g. death in the family).
- Perceived interference with social or personal relations.

- 'Sanctioning' – pressure from others to consult.
- 'Temporalizing of symptomatology' – e.g. 'If I feel the same way on Monday . . .' 'If I have another turn . . .'.

Practical
- Availability of resources (e.g. for consultation fees; childcare; transport).
- Access (availability of services and ability to get to them).
- Type, frequency, duration and severity of symptoms.
- Relative costs (e.g. wages lost through going to the GP's surgery; other trade-offs such as time).

Table 3.3 Advice or treatment in the popular sector: Northampton 1970 and 1985 (Source: Elliott-Binns, 1986).

	1970	1985
Patients attending GP who had received prior advice or treatment for their symptoms	96%	96%
Patients who had treated themselves prior to going to the doctor	55%	52%
Patients who had sought advice from their pharmacist	11%	16%

Beliefs about symptoms and their causes and how best to deal with them are often the most important aspect in decision-making about when to consult. They are, somewhat surprisingly, more important than the severity of symptoms in most cases. Indeed, there have been many studies showing how the decision to consult often takes place with no change in the severity or frequency of symptoms whatsoever. However, the prime trigger to consult is 'sanctioning' – this is observed in approximately 50% of decisions to consult. Those without pressure from others to consult are more likely to delay consulting and present when symptoms are more severe. Cultural and social beliefs are differentially distributed around the world. For example, studies conducted in the 1970s suggested that Italian-Americans in Boston were more likely to consult because of an interpersonal crisis or perceived interference with social or personal relations, while Irish-Americans were more likely to cite a perceived interference with a job or activity (e.g. sewing) and exhibit a temporalizing of symptomatology in their decision-making.

Table 3.3 is based on a study of 1000 patients attending a general practice in Northampton in 1970, and 500 patients attending in 1985. It indicates that most patients consult a GP after having received some kind of health care in the popular sector. The use of impersonal sources of advice, such as home doctor books, television and (currently, for those who can access it) the internet, is increasing. The use of home remedies is declining at about the same rate as people using the pharmacist is increasing.

The hierarchy of resort

In a situation of medical pluralism (Chapter 1) which pertains in most of the western world, the order in which people decide to use particular forms of therapy is known as the *hierarchy of resort*. In the UK the normal sector hierarchy is 'popular' (usually self-treatment), followed by 'professional' (e.g. GP), then 'folk' (if the professional's treatment doesn't work). In other societies the order may be different (e.g. self-treatment followed by 'folk healer' followed by 'professional'). Some people may try two or more sectors simultaneously (e.g. to cure their symptoms using western biomedicine, but deal with what is seen as the ultimate cause at the same time for example by using a faith healer).

Points of view

Why might a person decide to consult an alternative or complementary practitioner instead of a doctor?

The popular sector and the health professional

The recognition that vast amounts of health care take place in the popular sector without reference to a health care professional can be regarded as either threatening or fantastic. If it did not occur, the health service simply could not cope with the consequences. While acknowledging the problems that can arise from inappropriate advice from lay referral networks or self-medication, or the potential conflicts between self-help groups and the medical profession, the popular sector represents a resource that the wise doctor will respect and use to the patient's advantage. It is better to work with the sector and seek to understand it than to fight against and reject it. By acting in this way the good doctor can become a bridge between the different sectors of health care.

Ways in which a doctor can use the popular sector to the patient's (and carers') advantage

- Be sure to ask 'What have you done so far?'
- Give reassurance that the initial response to symptoms was understandable and/or appropriate, when someone does consult you.
- Provide advice about other options to help develop a patient's own resources for care.
- Recognize the value of self-help.
- Find out what self-help and other groups are available in the area.
- Compile a directory of local self-care resources.
- Alert patients to appropriate self-help groups in the area.
- Become involved in the recruitment, training and support of self-care trainers.
- Deliver some self-care training sessions, e.g. with suggestions for the management of short-term conditions.

Summary

- Vast amounts of health care activity takes place in the popular sector without reference to a health care professional.

- The family is one of the most important contexts for the maintenance of health and occurrence and treatment of illness.
- Most people do not live in a nuclear family. Recognizing the complexities of family life is important when providing a more holistic approach to health care.
- The pharmacist is an important element in the provision of self-care in the popular sector.
- Self-care often represents appropriate treatment and should be respected by a doctor when someone eventually consults them.
- Self-help groups are a growing area of health care, based on mutual aid, support and lobbying.
- The internet is increasingly important as a source of information and contact for people with a particular condition.
- Deciding to seek professional help (i.e. to consult) is affected by a complex interplay of social, psychological and practical factors. The most important of these appears to be 'sanctioning' – i.e. encouraging someone to consult.
- People often try different therapeutic options sequentially – the hierarchy of resort.
- It is important that a doctor understands how health and illness work outside the clinical context and use this knowledge to improve patient outcomes.

Further reading

Elliott-Binns, C. P. (1973) An analysis of lay medicine. *Journal of the Royal College of General Practitioners*, **23**: 255–64.

Elliott-Binns, C. P. (1986) An analysis of lay medicine: fifteen years later. *Journal of the Royal College of General Practitioners*, **36**: 542–4.

Lydeard, S. and Jones, R. (1989) Factors affecting the decision to consult with dyspepsia: comparison of consulters and non-consulters. *Journal of the Royal College of General Practitioners*, **39**: 495–8.

Pill, R. and Scott, N. (1982) Concepts of illness causation and responsibility: some preliminary data from a sample of working class mothers. *Social Science and Medicine*, **16**: 43–52.

Scambler, A., Scambler, G. and Craig, D. (1981) Kinship and friendship networks and women's demand for primary care. *Journal of the Royal College of General Practitioners*, **31**: 746–50.

Scambler, G. (2003) Health and illness behaviour. In G. Scambler (ed.) *Sociology as Applied to Medicine* (5th edn.). Edinburgh: Saunders.

Zola, I. (1973) Pathways to the doctor: from person to patient. *Social Science and Medicine*, **7**: 677–89.

Chapter 4

Health and health care in the professional sector

Introduction

The professional sector is the organized, politically dominant and legally sanctioned part of any health system, and in the UK is largely the domain of what we tend to call western scientific medicine (also known as biomedicine, cosmopolitan medicine or allopathic medicine). It includes all health care staff working in the sector, not just doctors. This chapter looks at the history of the growth of medicine to its dominant position in the UK, the knowledge base that enabled this to occur, its social organization and international variation. The professional sector, like the popular sector, is infused with cultural beliefs, attitudes and values. When we start to think of medicine as a cultural system in this way, with its singular ways of organizing itself and providing health care, it appears less universal in its form and functions than might initially be believed. Far from universal, western scientific medicine is culturally and historically specific, with differences in how it is practised both within and between health systems in different parts of the world. Medicine is not only a product of society, it also reflects that society's priorities and values. The National Health Service (NHS) as a way of organizing health care delivery

Lecture Notes: *The Social Basis of Medicine*, 1st edition. By Andrew Russell. Published 2009 by Blackwell Publishing. ISBN: 978-1-4051-3912-0

is unique to the UK. What is the future of health care in this country likely to be and what will be expected of our future doctors?

This chapter covers the following topics

The growth of medicine in the UK
The knowledge base of medicine
Social organization of medical practice in the UK
International variations in medical practice
The NHS as a unique way of organizing health care delivery

The growth of medicine in the UK

Reasons for the growth of western scientific medicine in the UK

- Legal sanctions and professional organization.
- Development of knowledge and the technological base.
- The efficacy of medical practice?

Legal sanctions and professional organization

In the eighteenth century, medicine was the domain of a variety of practitioners, among them physicians, barber-surgeons and apothecaries (see *Lecture Notes: Epidemiology and Public Health Medicine*, Chapter 18). There was much competition for patients, status and legitimacy. Physicians' training was relatively expensive and lengthy, and the Royal College of Physicians (founded in 1518) maintained something of a monopoly on the practice of medicine in cities such as London and Edinburgh. The medical journal *The Lancet*, founded by Thomas Wakeley in 1823, campaigned vigorously both against the elitism represented by the Colleges and against the work of unqualified 'quacks'. There was a clear need to distinguish between 'qualified' and 'unqualified' practitioners of all sorts (a dilemma still facing complementary and alternative medicines – see Chapter 5). In 1858, with the passage of the Medical Act, a national register of all physicians, surgeons and apothecaries was created, administered by the General Council of Medical Education and Registration (renamed the General Medical Council [GMC] in 1951). The British Medical Association (BMA) was formed in 1855 from an association created 20 years earlier to give voice to provincial practitioners; its journal, the *British Medical Journal*, was started in 1857. Over the next 100 years of so, an increasingly successful medical profession built up its independent power and public status. Branches of medicine proliferated and developed increasing specialization, while at the same time general practice became the cornerstone of primary health care delivery in the UK. While those who were not on the GMC's register were not barred from health care work, the register helped to establish the legitimacy of the medical profession and to differentiate scientific medicine from other forms of healing.

Development of knowledge and the technological base

The elevation in status of the medical profession would not have occurred without the developments in scientific knowledge and technology that transformed doctors' ability to diagnose and treat patients successfully. An example of these developments is the stethoscope, which originated in France in the early nineteenth century and subsequently developed its familiar 'two ear' shape in the US. This gave hitherto unimagined possibilities for auscultation of the thoracic cavity. Anatomical knowledge was also increasing dramatically – such was the demand for cadavers for use in medical training that 'resurrectionist' grave robbers (and murderers such as William Burke and William Hare in Edinburgh) provided bodies for private and public anatomy schools. Microscopes revealed bacteria to Louis Pasteur (working in France) and Robert Koch (in Germany) – just as the presence of viruses has been proved thanks to electron microscopes in the twentieth century. The development of thermometers (and x-ray technology in the twentieth century) added more tools to the doctor's diagnostic armoury. Developments in anaesthesia enabled much more complex surgical practices to begin. Later in the nineteenth century, Joseph Lister proved the value of antiseptic practices in preventing septicaemia in cases of compound fracture, evidence lending support to Pasteur's theories of bacterial infection.

The efficacy of medical practice?

While knowledge and technology were increasing during the nineteenth century, it is doubtful whether these changes had much impact on mortality until well into the twentieth century when, among other things, the development of antibiotics gave doctors something effective against acute bacterial infections. However, many of these illnesses (e.g. tuberculosis, cholera, measles, diphtheria) had started their decline long before any specific medical treatment was introduced. Improvements in the quality of life brought about through introduction of better sanitation, diet and hygiene practices were likely to have been much more significant than clinical interventions in reducing morbidity and mortality from these diseases.

The 1875 Public Health Act was a central government directive that consolidated earlier pieces of legislation. It obliged local authorities to provide clean water supplies and to appoint medical officers of health for every sanitary district in England and Wales. Although the impact of clinical medicine on morbidity and mortality in the nineteenth century was limited, the battles fought by medical officers of health up and down the country to improve the living conditions of ordinary people means that public health medicine can claim some credit for the reductions in the death rate that took place.

The knowledge base of medicine

The advances of nineteenth-century medicine were based on scientific method, involving the systematic investigation of all aspects of human anatomy and physiology. Chapter 1 considered the contrast between the biomedical and the biopsychosocial approaches in medicine. There has been considerable diversification of views through time, but the medical worldview remains grounded in particular broad scientific principles that form the knowledge base of the discipline (Table 4.1).

The empirical approach of scientific medicine has yielded some excellent results in the treatment of physical illnesses, but until recently it tended to be much less effective in dealing with mental illness (see Chapter 9). This is partly because the definition of mental 'illness' depends

much more on behaviour (and what is 'normal' behaviour is much harder to assess than what is 'normal' physiology), and partly because, until recently, less was known about the biology of the brain/nervous system than of many other body systems.

While the approach of medicine to causation has been described as proximalist, clinical medicine often has no time to deal with causes at all, except where there is a therapeutic reason for doing so (e.g. knowing what has been ingested when a patient presents with a drug overdose). 'Bad luck' is perhaps accepted as a wider category of causation in biomedicine than in the societies it serves, and this leads to patients seeking explanations (and solutions) for ill health that go beyond 'bad luck' (e.g. Why me? Why now?) that take them beyond the realms of clinical medical treatment.

The notion of 'evidence'

In recent years evidence-based medicine (EBM) has challenged the validity of 'experience' *per se* as a means of decision-making about how to treat

Table 4.1 The knowledge base of medicine.

Principle	Meaning	Comments
Empiricism	Based on experience, i.e. use of the senses to explore and analyse the real world	Contrasts with speculation without direct observation or adherence to 'perfect knowledge' contained in ancient texts (e.g. in Indian Ayurveda) Fundamental to understanding symptomatology and diagnostics
Proximalism	In explaining ill health, tendency to focus on proximal, immediate causes (e.g. smoking)	Ultimate causes (which may be social or economic) tend to be disregarded
Physicalism	Nature conceived of in mainly physical terms. 'Machine view' of the body, its anatomy and physiology	Fundamental to therapeutic interventions, mainly by surgical or pharmaceutical methods
Generalizability	Aims for 'one treatment/many people' In developing any pharmaceutical product, the 'active ingredient' is always sought that will work for large populations	Contrasts with 'one person/many treatments' in (e.g.) Chinese medicine, where the synergy of different products working together is tested on the individual
Modernism	Belief that medicine is constantly progressing in a linear fashion, leading to constant refinement of knowledge	'Old-fashioned' theories and treatments redundant

the individual patient. Based on population-based research and clinical trials, it aims to provide up-to-date, definitive information about 'what works' and provides benefit, and what does not. Knowledge in EBM is graded according to its rigour and robustness, with the systematic review of randomized controlled trials at the top of the tree and case reports at the bottom (see *Lecture Notes: Epidemiology and Public Health Medicine*, Chapter 11, p. 82). Doctors are kept up to date concerning treatments through the compilation of 'best evidence' in protocols and guidelines.

However, only 10–20% of medical practice has been subject to randomized controlled trials, and much of the rest is unlikely to be, due to cost, time and ethical issues. While few would question that it is preferable for doctors to use EBM rather than out-of-date textbooks acquired in medical school, EBM poses challenges for other principles in medicine such as patient choice and clinical experience. GPs have to bear the brunt of these dilemmas, and also the bulk of the guidelines and protocols that are produced, due to their 'generalist' status. Guidelines are intended to provide doctors with information in an easily assimilable form to enable gold standard, evidence based care. However, recent studies have indicated that there is a danger of GPs becoming swamped by a plethora of EBM guidelines. Education programmes involving outreach visits, particularly if this person is recognized as an opinion leader in the field, are frequently necessary to establish their validity and use. New IT packages in general practice are designed to ensure prescribing is referenced to guidelines as far as possible. Yet while many regard guidelines as a useful tool, most would agree that clinical consultation and practice are not simply a matter of applying scientific evidence to the individual patient.

Case study: Use of guidelines for the treatment of hypertension in elderly patients

In 1998 a study found that GPs were under-treating cases of hypertension by as much as 50%. Good management of hypertension is one of the best and most cost-effective ways of preventing the misery and mortality risks associated with heart disease and stroke. Yet despite being aware of the risks posed by hypertension in the elderly and the benefits of its treatment, fewer than half the GPs were complying with the broad recommendations of evidence-based guidelines. Why?

GPs in a study in Merseyside who were the subjects of an educational intervention to improve the management of hypertension in the elderly expressed doubts about the applicability of trial data to particular patients. Many demonstrated poor adherence to practice protocols and some exhibited ageist attitudes regarding who they considered merited treatment. For others, time pressure and financial considerations made it a low priority, as did the absence of effective IT systems and educational mentors.

Case study: *Helicobacter pylori* as a paradigm shift in medicine

In 1982, J. Robin Warren and Barry Marshall, two medical researchers working in Western Australia, identified a micro-organism, *Helicobacter pylori*, associated with inflammation of the mucosa of the stomach lining, particularly in and around ulcer craters. It took a year to isolate and culture the bacteria successfully, after which, in order to prove the association between *H. pylori* and stomach problems, Warren and Marshall tested the cultures on themselves by ingesting them. Both developed gastritis, but not ulcers. In fact, subsequent epidemiological studies, while proving an association between *H. pylori* infection and stomach ulcers (95% of people in the UK with duodenal ulcer have *H. pylori* infection), found only one fifth of the 35% of people in the UK with *H. pylori* infection developed ulcers. Marshall's findings were first reported in 1984 and updated in a later study published in *The Lancet* in 1988, where he suggested that a mix of antibiotics and bismuth (the so-called 'triple therapy') cured 92% of ulcers.

The research into *H. pylori* was widely derided at first since it flew in the face of medical orthodoxy. Prior to Warren and Marshall's work, microscopists had frequently observed the curved bacteria on their stomach mucosa slides, but their presence was attributed to artefact or post-mortem contamination. After all, everyone knew bacteria could not live in the acidic environment of the stomach. Ulcers were caused by excess acid in the gastric mucosa generally

(continued on p. 40)

(continued)

attributed to stress, personality type or upbringing. Such a psychosomatic model of ulcer formation was totally at odds with the infective agent view that the Australians were proposing. Ten years after Marshall's initial work, 27% of gastroenterologists in the UK responding to a postal survey still did not consider *H. pylori* to be the cause of duodenal ulcers.

The *H. pylori* story is a good demonstration of a paradigm shift in medicine – findings that transform our understanding of (in this case) the microbiology and pathology of the stomach. The fact that such a shift took place is hardly surprising, given the evidence that Warren and Marshall put together. What is interesting is how steadfast so many experts in the field were in their disbelief about the role of *H. pylori* for so long. While the fact that the majority of people with *H. pylori* infection do not develop ulcers might have been a confounding factor and could still suggest a stress-related 'trigger', the fact that 95% of people with duodenal ulcers had *H. pylori* infection and that eradicating the infection cured the ulcers in the majority of cases should have alerted the sceptics to something. As it was, in 1993 only 25% of gastroenterologists were using the triple therapy for an ulcer at first presentation and 17% never used it.

Social organization of medical practice in the UK

It is helpful to think of the professional sector in the UK as consisting of a set of interlinked but distinct social groups, each with its own priorities, values, history and ways of doing things. As a result, each also has different ways of relating to other health professional groups and to the general public.

Paramedics
Prosthetists and orthotists
Radiographers
Speech and language therapists
Medical social workers
Counsellors

Far from being equal members of a team, the relative status of the groups is hotly contested. In addition, there are subgroups (and hence subcultures) within many of the larger groups. Nurses make up the single largest category of health professionals in the NHS (over 315,000 in 2004) and include practice nurses, nurse practitioners, district nurses, community psychiatric nurses and school nurses as well as the hierarchy of nurses found in hospital settings. 'Doctors' is also a category that covers a diverse range of subgroups, each with its own history and ways of approaching practice.

Health professionals in the UK

Doctors
Nurses
Midwives
Health visitors
Social workers
Physiotherapists
Occupational therapists
Pharmacists
Dieticians
Opticians
Dentists
Hospital technicians
Nursing auxiliaries
Medical receptionists
Clinical psychologists
Educational psychologists
Arts therapists
Biomedical scientists
Chiropodists/podiatrists
Clinical scientists

Medical specialities in the UK (by college membership qualification)

Clinical specialities
Medicine (Member of the Royal College of Physicians – MRCP)
  accident and emergency
  general medicine

geriatrics
cardiology
neurology
respiratory
endocrinology
rheumatology
gastroenterology
renal (nephrology)
genitourinary
dermatology
haematology
oncology and radiotherapy
occupational health
public health
pharmacology and therapeutics
palliative

Surgery (Fellow of the Royal College of Surgeons – FRCS)
general
urology
orthopaedics
neurosurgery
plastic and reconstruction surgery
cardiothoracic
vascular
ear, nose and throat

General Practice (Member of the Royal College of General Practitioners – MRCGP)

Ophthalmology (Member of the Royal College of Ophthalmologists – MRCOphth)

Paediatrics and Child Health (Member of the Royal College of Paediatrics and Child Health – MRCPCH)
general
neonatology

Obstetrics and Gynaecology (Member of the Royal College of Obstetrics and Gynaecology – MRCOG)
foetal medicine

Psychiatry (Member of the Royal College of Psychiatrists – MRCPsych)

Anaesthetics (Fellow of the Royal College of Anaesthesiologists – FRCA)

Service specialities

Pathology (Member of the Royal College of Pathologists – MRCPath)
microbiology
histopathology
haematology
biochemistry

Diagnostic imaging (Fellow of the Royal College of Radiologists – FRCR)

As medicine has developed, so have the variety and complexity of the specialities. Many of the elements in the list above overlap, for example:

• A haematologist may well combine laboratory with clinical work, as in the blood transfusion service.

• Accident and emergency medicine combines medicine and surgery.

• Many 'general' physicians in the hospital service provide expertise across a broad area, including at least some aspects of gastroenterology, respiratory medicine, cardiology, endocrinology and nephrology.

• General practice covers all the major clinical specialities listed above, in primary care settings.

There are also some interesting anomalies, for example:

• Although endocrinology is the study of hormones, the organs from which they originate and the diseases associated with them, many endocrinologists do not deal with diabetes mellitus, which is one of the most common endocrine disorders.

• Although listed as a clinical speciality, public health rarely involves consultations with patients, being much more population-based in its approach. Nearly one quarter of public health specialists working at consultant level in the UK are not medical doctors.

• Reflecting their different historical origins, consultant surgeons are addressed as 'Mr', whereas all other consultants are addressed as 'Dr'.

Medicine is also represented by diverse institutions such as hospitals, clinics and professional bodies. Every institution is unique, fuelled by the dynamics of the individuals working within it, their interactions and socialization as a group, its environmental context and available resources. An institutional culture can be positive, where good team work contributes positively to better care of patients, or negative, as in the case of the paediatric cardiac unit of the Bristol Royal Infirmary (BRI).

Case study: The Bristol Royal Infirmary

The Bristol Royal Infirmary inquiry was established by the government in 1998 following concerns expressed about the high mortality rates among infants receiving complex cardiac surgical services at the BRI between 1984 and 1995. It reported its findings in 2001. The report demonstrated that between 1991 and 1995 between 30 and 35 more children aged under one year died after open heart surgery at the BRI than was typical of similar heart units elsewhere in England. This was not found to be due to differences in the severity of the cases. While mortality rates fell throughout the rest of the country, as time went on this did not happen at the BRI. Although concerns about standards of open heart surgery were first raised in 1986, no one acted effectively to tackle the problems. The report criticized the protective 'club culture' (by which was meant an old-school 'gentleman's club') of the consultants which led to a failure to identify and acknowledge that problems existed. It was an anaesthetist 'whistle-blower' who finally set in motion the chain of events that led to the suspension of children's heart surgery at the BRI in 1995. Since then many changes have taken place nationally in how medical practice is monitored.

Medicine as a reflection of society

Medicine is not only partly a product of the society in which it is located, it also reflects that society (Chapter 1). For example, the predominant roles of men and women are reflected in the distribution of the sexes within the professional sector. In the UK in 2002, 78% of people working in the NHS were women. The majority of them were working in what are generally regarded as the lower levels of the service, as cleaners, caterers, ancillary workers and nurses. The title 'nurse' alludes to maternal nurturance, and over 90% of nurses are women, although a disproportionate number of male nurses (30–40%) occupy senior nursing management positions. The relationships of doctors, nurses and patients can be seen as mirroring the gender divisions of the nineteenth-century Victorian family: doctor = father, nurse = mother and patient = child. The nurse's sphere remains separate from and subordinate to that of the doctor. Until recently, UK hospital nurses were still known by gender-linked family titles ('sister'; 'matron'). The nurse is intimately involved with the patient's body, including its waste products. Hospital doctors, by contrast, spend relatively little time caring for patients, dealing rather with specialized knowledge about the inner workings of their patients' bodies.

As we move up through the status hierarchy of medicine, the number of women declines (Figure 4.1). In the UK in 2002, 43% of junior hospital doctors (registrars, senior house officers and house officers) were women; just over 20% of women were consultants. However, the lower proportion of women in more senior grades partly reflects a history of lower female entry into medical schools. The male:female ratio among medical school entrants reached 50:50 in 1991. By 2002, 61% of UK medical and dentistry students were women, and the entry of women that year was 64%.

In contrast to the entry into medical school, the *largest* percentage of women consultants under the age of 45 in the UK in 2002 was in geriatrics (37.7%). This was equivalent to the increasing proportion of women GPs; in 2002 nearly 60% of GP registrars were women. By 2005, 40% of GPs were women, half of whom worked part-time (compared with 12% of male GPs). Some medical specialties, arguably those that occupy the 'highest status' niches in medicine, such as neurology, cardiology and other surgical specialties, continue to be male-dominated; and far fewer women enter the surgical professions compared to the numbers that enter medical school.

Case study: The woman in the surgeon's body?

An anthropologist spent two years studying male and female surgeons in the US and elsewhere, during which time she made some interesting observations and recorded some illuminating statements. She found that female surgeons faced attitudinal barriers in the workplace that may be significant in explaining why success as a female surgeon is particularly hard to achieve.

Situation: Operating theatre of a world famous cancer centre
Characters: 'Sir James', an aristocratic surgeon (male); his first assistant (female)
Event: During the procedure, a male medical student flattered Sir James on the elegance of his technique. 'Yes', he replied, 'but surgery is *never* elegant when there are women in the room.'
Outcome: Comment passes unchallenged.

The comment is particularly noteworthy because clearly there are almost always women in the operating theatre, such as nurses (normally female) and maybe a female anaesthesiologist. What was significant to Sir James was the presence of a woman in a higher role, as his first assistant.

Situation: Emergency situation in transplant operation
Characters: Chief resident transplant surgeon (female); hospital telephone operator (female)
Event: Hospital operator being 'obtuse and obstructive'. Chief resident explodes 'Goddamit, someone's dying, get me Dr so-and-so!'
Outcome: Operator files a complaint with chief of surgery.

The event is noteworthy because of the many examples where male surgeons display impatience – it is most unlikely a man would have been sanctioned for (merely) swearing in this way.

Situation: Operating theatre
Characters: Surgeon (male); nurses (female)
Event: Surgeon throws a tantrum (known as a 'doctor fit')
Outcome: Surgeon is later described by nurses as 'temperamental' or 'highly strung'. Nurses later joke about him behind his back, but in the operating theatre they pay scrupulous attention, as if the surgeon is a volatile substance that might explode at any time if they make a wrong or tardy move.

Situation: Operating theatre
Characters: Surgeon (female); nurses (female)
Event: Surgeon throws a tantrum
Outcome: Nurses label surgeon 'a bitch'. Nurses become slow and sulky in the face of female tantrums. A slow operation poses a greater risk to the patient.

The striking comparison of these vignettes highlights the problems women surgeons have not just with superiors but with female nursing subordinates. This is in addition to the problems they face juggling domestic commitments with their high-pressure careers. They are perceived as, and have to work extra hard to counteract the perception that they are, 'the wrong body in the wrong place'.

One explanation for the discrepancy in numbers between, say, general practice and surgery is that women 'look and act right' for general practice, while it is men who 'look and act right' for surgery. Traditional gender roles in the UK tend to stereotype women as more nurturing and expressive, and less technically skilful, than men. Hence they are relatively under-represented in surgery. Of course, there may be other practical reasons for this discrepancy, such as more opportunities for part-time working in general practice (at consultant level, more women than men work part-time). There may be indirect influences, such as some degree of bias in those who advise women on career choices, and the opportunities that are made available to women as the progress in their careers. Finally, the situation may be an expression of women's true preferences and individual freedom of choice.

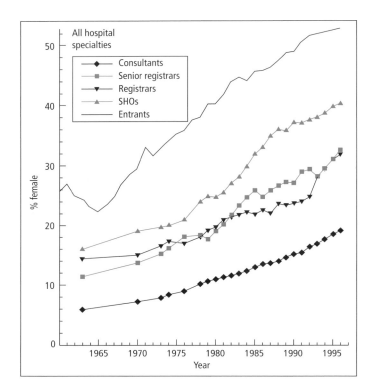

Figure 4.1 Proportion of female medical school entrants and female doctors at various stages of hospital careers for the years 1963 to 1996 (Source: McManus and Sproston, 2000).

As the gender relationships between the sexes change (or perhaps because of a changing sense of vocation towards medicine) men are increasingly selecting part-time work or are expressing their intent to do so. Such shifts at the individual level can, in aggregate, have major implications for workforce planning. A possible result of the increased opportunities for flexible and part-time working (for women and men) is a reduction in continuity of patient care, a fragmentation of the contribution of individuals (especially in the domain of medical leadership) and increased difficulty in effective team working.

International variations in medical practice

The practice of medicine varies not only within health systems but between them. Given its scientific credentials, which are generally (wrongly) assumed to be universal, we might expect medi-

cine would be practised in a standard way across continents. However, as anyone who has experienced medical practice in other countries can testify, medicine is extremely variable in its manifestations. One obvious reason is the different level of resources available in different countries. Environment and geography undoubtedly play a part too, if only because the types and presentation of diseases vary sometimes according to genetic and environmental differences as well as distance from medical services. However, when one looks at countries which are broadly comparable socio-economically, environmentally and genetically, it can be seen that cultural differences are as important as socio-economic ones in explaining the differences in medical practice internationally. Medicine is not only the product of its society, it also reflects and is part of the cultural systems of that society.

There are two main reasons for international variations in medical practice to consider in more detail: resource levels and cultural differences in the way medicine is practised.

Resource levels

While resource issues clearly have a major part to play in explaining the wide variation in the figures shown in Table 4.2 (Nepal compared to the UK, for example) there may well be other, cultural factors to take into account. We should also question whether physical measures such as number of doctors or hospital beds actually imply anything about the quality of the services provided.

Table 4.2 Doctors and hospital beds per 1000 population in selected countries.

Country	Doctors per 1000 population (year of data collection)	Hospital beds per 1000 population (year of data collection)
China	1.06 (2001)	2.3 (2004)
Egypt	0.54 (2003)	2.2 (2003)
Germany	3.37 (2003)	7.6 (2004)
Jamaica	0.85 (2003)	1.8 (2004)
Japan	1.98 (2002)	12.9 (2001)
Nepal	0.21 (2004)	0.2 (2001)
Pakistan	0.74 (2004)	0.7 (2003)
UK	2.3 (1997)	4.0 (2003)
US	2.56 (2000)	3.3 (2003)

Source: WHO (2006)

Hospital beds in the UK – is less more?

Between 1984 and 2004, the number of hospital beds in the UK fell by almost a third, from 221,617 to 145,218, although the number of patients needing to stay overnight increased by 57% during the same period (and day cases increased by 341%). There is no evidence that patient satisfaction with the service they received in hospital decreased at all during this period. The report in which these data were presented queried the value of assessing service provision by means of resource indicators such as number of beds. Various reasons were suggested to explain the reduction in bed numbers:

Patients being treated at home – e.g. new chemotherapy treatments can be administered to patients in their own home.

Care being more effectively provided elsewhere – e.g. doctors in local surgeries carrying out minor surgery.

Technology changing the type of treatment needed (and hence length of recovery time) – e.g. keyhole surgery has a shorter recovery time so patients can be discharged earlier.

Improvements in chronic disease management – e.g. a self-treatment plan for people with chronic bronchitis helps them manage their condition and reduces the number of emergency admissions to hospital.

Changes to emergency care reducing admissions to hospital – e.g. emergency care practitioners in the ambulance service treating people in their own home.

Reduced waiting times for discharge from hospitals – e.g. reducing the need for patients to wait for the weekly consultant's ward round before discharge.

On the other hand, in certain sectors the reduction in the number of beds has led to shortages and reduced services, e.g. the provision of emergency beds for acute psychiatric care.

Cultural differences in the way medicine is practised

Japan has an astonishing number of hospital beds (see above) – more than three times as many as the UK. Such a large difference is not due to socio-economic factors. Hospital stays in Japan tend to be much longer than in other countries and include convalescence periods that are spent at home in the UK. For example, in Japan women normally spend 5–7 days in hospital after a trouble-free vaginal delivery and three weeks after a Caesarean section. This compares with average stays of 1.4 days and 3.4 days respectively for the same procedures in the UK. In a country with fewer holidays and a reluctance among office staff to take holidays, hospital stays are regarded by some people in Japan as an alternative to a vacation.

Medical practice in Japan – some differences

Appointments – to see a doctor, normal practice is to go early in the morning and queue for attendance on a 'first come, first served' basis. People feel more comfortable without an appointment.

Surrogate patients – the illness of one family member is the concern of all, and it is quite acceptable for a friend or relative to substitute for the patient either by taking over interactions with the doctor (with the patient present) or by coming in place of the patient (e.g. for repeat prescriptions).

Attitudes to cancer – if a patient is diagnosed with cancer, it is generally regarded as best policy not to tell him or her because the demoralization such knowledge would cause could undermine efforts to overcome the disease.

All these are graphic indications of the role of culture in the way services are organized and delivered. However, even comparison of three Anglo-American countries indicates significant differences in medical practice (Table 4.3).

Various hypotheses were proposed to explain these differences (Table 4.4).

The inconsistent figures for resources suggest that these did not appear to be significant in explaining the cross-national differences in surgery rates during the decade. The Gross National Product (GNP) spent on health care is to a certain extent a reflection of national priorities and values and correlates with surgical rates. New techniques introduced in North America, but not England and Wales, during the decade do appear to be significant, but perhaps more so are the treatment styles and philosophies of patient management – the technological imperative that if one has a technology or technique, then one should use it. These both reflect prevalent cultural attitudes (Figure 4.2).

Table 4.3 Surgical rates in the US, Canada, and England and Wales, 1966–76.

	US	Canada	England and Wales
Overall surgery rates	Highest of the three countries; increased by 25% over the decade to become 125% higher than England and Wales rates at the end	60% higher than in England and Wales throughout decade	Remained constant, lowest of the three
Caesarean sections Hysterectomy	12% in 1976 Double the rate for England and Wales throughout decade	12% in 1976 Double the rate for England and Wales throughout the decade	7% in 1976

Table 4.4 Hypotheses to explain differences in the way services are organized and delivered.

Hypothesis	Indicators	Comments
Resources	Number of beds	US operative rates 40% greater than Canada, yet Canada had 30% more beds than the US
	Surgeons per capita	Increased in both Canada and England and Wales
Health profile	Mortality rates	No significant differences
National priorities	GNP spend on health care (1970)	England and Wales 5% Canada 7% USA 9%
Technology	New techniques	Increases in specialist cardiac, vascular and thoracic surgery in Canada and the US during the decade
Culture	Treatment styles Philosophies of patient management	Significant differences observed

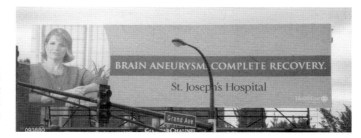

Figure 4.2 Billboard in St Paul, MN. Advertising individual hospitals in this way and in such a manner is virtually unheard of in the UK, and thus tells us a lot about the culture of medicine in the US (Source: author).

Case study: James Cook University Hospital, Middlesbrough, UK – a cultural resource?

When James Cook University Hospital (JCUH) opened in Middlesbrough in 2001 it was the largest tertiary care hospital in Europe. (The 'James Cook' title was chosen to represent the connectedness of the hospital to its community: the famous eighteenth-century explorer James Cook was born in the area.) The new hospital contained a number of artworks especially commissioned to reflect the Cook theme and were intended by the Hospital Trust to help provide a pleasant and soothing 'therapeutic environment' for patients and staff alike. However, they were also explicitly intended to signal that the JCUH was a high-quality building reflecting (according to the architects) 'the aspirations of the Middlesbrough community' (Figures 4.3 and 4.4).

Middlesbrough is one of the most deprived towns in England and the government's new hospital building programme is intended to contribute to urban regeneration and renewal by instilling a sense of community and civic pride. According to government regulations, 1% of hospital build costs must be devoted to art installations. The striking thing about the arts programme at JCUH was that publicity about it not only targeted patients and staff, but also members of the wider community who were invited to the hospital to see the artworks and to attend concerts in the hospital atrium.

How should hospital building funds be distributed? Should a hospital be purely a functional building, like a factory, or should it be embellished and decorated, and if so with what, and why? Should hospitals become more of a 'cultural resource' for the whole community?

(continued on p. 48)

(continued)

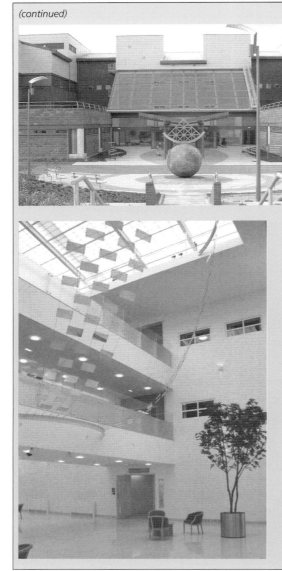

Figure 4.3 Main entrance to JCUH, Middlesbrough, showing globe and sextant sculpture signifying the journeys of James Cook around the world (Source: CAHHM, Durham).

Figure 4.4 The atrium, JCUH, showing commissioned glasswork. The glasswork is meant to represent the sails of Cook's boat, but one visitor interpreted it as being tiles from the space shuttle *Challenger* disaster! (Source: CAHHM, Durham).

The NHS as a unique way of organizing health care delivery

The NHS is the main employment destination of medical students in the UK. Since its foundation in 1948, costs have escalated. The 5% of GDP spent on health care in 1970 has risen to 7.7% (£69 billion in 2005) and is now higher, proportionately, than that of the US, where health spending as a proportion of GDP has declined. The UK government intends to increase this expenditure further, up to £92 billion in 2007/8, so that spending on health will be equivalent to the average for the EU. Most of the expenditure is on hospital services, of which 65% is spent on salaries: 1.3 million people are employed by the NHS, which makes it not only the largest UK employer (5% of the total UK workforce) but one of the largest employers in the world. Clearly, the NHS is an important factor in the economy as well as in the country's health. It is also an important plank of government policy and hence risks becoming something of a political football or 'hot potato'. From its brave beginnings in 1948 when it was stated 'it will provide you with all medical, dental and nursing care . . . There are no charges, except for a few special items', some charges have been introduced, particularly in the field of dental health services, optician services and prescribing. However, the cost of a prescription (in 2008, £7.10) is far less than the cost of many of the pharmaceuticals prescribed, and 75% of people do not pay prescription charges at all. For all the criticisms of it, the NHS is still admired throughout the world as a unique and efficient means of providing good health care, and most people in the UK are pleased that we have 'the good old NHS'.

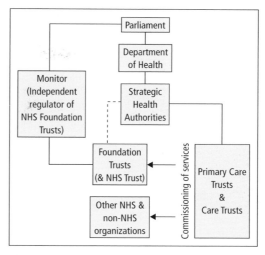

Figure 4.5 The structure of the NHS in England, 2007.

In the NHS in 2005, each week there were

- 1.4 million people who received NHS help in their home.
- More than 800,000 treated in hospital outpatient clinics.
- 700,000 who visited an NHS dentist.
- Over 10,000 babies delivered.
- Over 150,000 pairs of feet inspected.
- Over 50,000 emergency ambulance journeys.
- 500,000 telephones calls to NHS Direct (and a similar number of internet connections).
- 3 million people who visited their GP.
- 8.5 million items dispensed on NHS prescriptions.
- Around 1200 hip operations, 3000 heart operations and 1050 kidney operations.

Structure of the NHS

The NHS is in a state of constant revolution – some have said disruptive governance – which means that its structures and organizational diagrams change with alarming regularity. Devolution has also changed the arrangements for health care, with the four countries that comprise the UK developing their own structures. The current structure of the NHS in England is shown in Figure 4.5.

Department of Health

The Department of Health (DoH) is intended to give strategic leadership to the NHS and social care organizations. The objectives of the DoH include:

- To provide health improvement and health protection services for the population of England.
- To enhance the quality and safety of services, including faster access and more choice.
- To improve capacity and efficiency of the services.
- To reform the system.

The DoH is headed by the Secretary of State for Health, who is accountable to Parliament for the functioning of the NHS. The Secretary works with five Ministers for Health, and the NHS Chief Executive and Permanent Secretary. The latter chairs the DoH Management Board, whose members include the Chief Medical Officer, together with a number of national Clinical Directors, clinical experts in their field who oversee implementation of the NHS Plan for their specialities.

The NHS Plan

The NHS Plan was first introduced in 2000 as a ten-year programme of improvement and development. The NHS Plan had many aims, among which were to increase capacity, reduce waiting times and improve the quality of clinical services. Strategies to implement the NHS Plan have included the following.

National Service Frameworks
National Service Frameworks (NSFs) are designed to:
* Set national standards and define the way a service should be provided.
* Put in practice strategies to support implementation.
* Establish performance milestones against which progress within an agreed timescale can be measured.
* Form one of a range of measures to raise quality and decrease variations of service in the NHS.
Each NSF is developed with the assistance of an external reference group made up of health professionals, service users, carers, health service managers and other agencies. NSFs currently exist for nine subject areas:
* Mental Health 1999
* Coronary Heart Disease 2000
* National Cancer plan 2000
* Older people 2001
* Diabetes 2001
* Children's services 2004
* Renal Service part 1 2004, part 2 2005
* Long-term conditions 2005
* Chronic Obstructive Pulmonary Disease 2008

Priorities and Planning Frameworks
Since the publication of the NHS Plan, the Department of Health has increasingly focused national priorities on a limited number of targets. These were published in the Priorities and Planning Framework and have been updated annually. Those for 2005–8 were for the NHS to:
* Deliver a financial surplus.
* Achieve health inequalities targets, e.g. reduction in mortality rates from heart disease, stroke, reducing smoking rates, reduction in mortality rates from cancer.
* Achieve a maximum 31-day wait from referral to diagnosis and a 62-day wait from diagnosis to treatment for patients referred urgently with a diagnosis of suspected cancer.
* Ensure that by 2008 no one waits more than 18 weeks from GP referral to treatment of any sort.
* Achieve a year-on-year reduction in MRSA infections.
* Ensure that all hospital appointments are booked via the Choose and Book system and patients are offered a choice of at least four providers.
* Ensure that by 2008 all patients referred to a genitourinary clinic have an appointment within 48 hours.
These are the top priorities which Primary Care Trusts, as commissioners of services, will need to achieve. In the guide it is stressed that there will be less scope for new initiatives. This is an important point since proposed developments outside the national priorities will have a limited chance of being successful.

NHS performance ratings and annual health check
Between 2001 and 2005 the DoH published NHS performance ratings in which NHS organizations in England were allocated a rating of 0, 1, 2 or 3 stars. From March 2005 the star rating was replaced by an 'annual health check', organized by the Healthcare Commission, which is based on quality of services and use of resources.

Managed Clinical Networks
These provide clinical services that are delivered by clinical networks covering more than one Trust.

Strategic Health Authorities

There are ten Strategic Health Authorities (SHAs) in England, each covering a population of between 2.5 and 7.5 million with boundaries that are, with one exception, coterminous with a Government Office. The main roles of the SHAs are:
- To ensure coherency and to develop strategies for improving the health service in their region (or 'patch').
- To manage performance of the region's local health services (with the exception of the Foundation Trusts) on behalf of the DoH.
- To build capacity in the regional NHS and below.
- To ensure that national priorities are integrated into local health plans.

Primary Care Trusts

Primary Care Trusts (PCTs) are the cornerstone of the NHS in England. Funding for hospitals (NHS Trusts and Foundation Trusts) and contracts with non-NHS providers now come primarily from PCTs. Each PCT covers a population of approximately 150,000–300,000, and is responsible for:
- Planning and securing services, by determining which health services the local population needs and ensuring their provision. This is done by commissioning the volume and quality of services provided by the PCT itself, hospital and other providers.
- Improving the health of the community.
- Integrating health and social care locally by ensuring that NHS organizations work in partnership with Local Authorities.

Care Trusts

Care Trusts are NHS bodies that work in both health and social care. They can be established when NHS organizations and Local Authorities agree to work together; their functions are determined by this partnership. At present only a small number of Care Trusts have been established, although their numbers are expected to increase in the future. In places where Care Trusts have not been established, PCTs and Social Services work as independent agencies.

Foundation Trusts

Foundation Trusts are a relatively new development (first established in April 2004). They are freestanding organizations constituted as independent, non-profit-making organizations. Foundation Trusts are owned by their members who are local people, employees and other key stakeholders. The Secretary of State for Health does not have the power to direct NHS Foundation Trusts and is not involved in appointing board members. Instead, Monitor, the independent regulator, issues licences for the Foundation Trusts to operate and is accountable to Parliament for ensuring that the terms of the licence are upheld. Licences cover a number of areas:
- Delivery of care to NHS patients.
- The clinical services which it must provide to the local community.
- Participation in the education and development of health care staff in the NHS.
- The financial arrangements under which it must operate.
- The Trust's relationship with other NHS and Social Care bodies and use of IT.

Foundation Trusts are also subject to inspection by the Healthcare Commission and are accountable to PCTs through the contractual arrangements they make with them.

NHS Trusts

NHS Trusts continue to run some hospitals and are accountable to Strategic Health Authorities, but are rapidly being phased out by the DoH and turned into Foundation Trusts.

Other NHS and non-NHS organizations

Other types of NHS provider and non-NHS organizations have an increasingly important role to play in implementing government policy to increase capacity and provide more care closer to patients' homes, in community facilities rather than acute hospitals. Outpatient and day case surgery work are particularly targeted for this approach. Among the areas of medicine affected are:

- Dermatology.
- Ear, Nose and Throat.
- General Surgery.
- Orthopaedics.
- Urology.
- Gynaecology.

A number of other organizations are now delivering health care. These include:

Clinical Assessment, Treatment and Support Services (CATS) – operated either by the NHS or the independent sector. GP referrals are assessed in these centres before being referred to hospital or to another GP with a specialist interest, another provider or another part of the CATS service. This new approach may have a significant impact on the number of referrals hospitals receive.

Treatment centres – operated either by the NHS or more usually by the independent sector. These are stand-alone organizations usually providing elective diagnostics and surgery in areas such as radiology and endoscopy.

Primary care centres – being developed by a increasing number of PCTs to provide services such as

clinics, urgent care as an alternative to Accident and Emergency Departments for non-trauma patients, renal dialysis and endoscopy.

Independent hospitals – NHS patients are increasingly being referred to independent hospitals for NHS care.

Social enterprise ventures – these are organizations that are run along business lines but where any profits made are reinvested in the community or service developments. These are part of the third sector (non-NHS, non-independent sector). The DoH is encouraging the formation of this type of organization through dedicated funding as a way of delivering innovative health and social care. The types of services that these organizations provide include alcohol and substance misuse programmes, services for vulnerable adults and other community-based services. Voluntary organizations and charities may run them. The long-term viability of these types of organizations is as yet unknown.

The future

It is impossible to say what the NHS will be like in ten years' time. We can, however, make predictions about the health and health care challenges it will face.

Some health and health care challenges for the NHS in the twenty-first century

- Rebalancing the NHS – from a sickness to a health service (i.e. from diagnosis, treatment and salvage work to predictions and management/risk modification).
- Continuing upward trend in demand from people suffering from chronic illness and long-term health conditions.
- Public health keen to concentrate on 'upstream' rather than 'downstream' issues.
- Changing role of hospitals (from big to community).
- Increasing role of informatics.
- Spiralling costs due to:
    Increasingly sophisticated technology.
    Rising incomes and their impact on the NHS's salary bill.
    Increased demand for health services and greater expectations about what it will provide.
    Increasing numbers of patients over 65.
    Payback for large-scale Private Finance Initiative (PFI) construction projects carried out since 1997 (at an average cost of 30% more than public sector borrowing and work).
- Pressure for greater patient/public involvement in and responsibility for health and health care.
- Multidisciplinary team working.
- Community care using non-clinical organizations and services.
- Ever-present possibility of the arrival of a 'superbug'.

Some of the ways in which these challenges can be met include the use of health trainers, a new category of professional proposed in by the 2005 government White Paper *Choosing Health*. The idea is that these trainers will engage in health promotion work with people in the community. Their tasks will largely concern lifestyle issues such as smoking, alcohol abuse, exercise and healthy eating, although in some circumstances their scope could be wider. Open access services and 'walk-in' clinics will assist in changing the role of hospitals as well as control costs to a certain extent. While the costs of new treatments are generally high, the cost of existing treatments tends to fall. An example of this is the use of statins to control high blood cholesterol, one of which (simvastatin 10 mg) has been available OTC since July 2004. Making more medicines available OTC is part of the trend towards giving the public greater responsibility for looking after their own health care needs. Other examples include patient-centred clinical practice, which enables participation in decision-making about health care. 'Expert patients' (particularly those with long-term conditions) can also contribute to service delivery and participate in service planning (see Chapter 12).

Case study: Private health care in the UK

While everyone is entitled to health care that is free at point of delivery in the UK, a significant proportion of the population pay for private medical care, either as one-off payments to a private doctor or hospital or by purchasing private medical insurance. There are currently 15 private health insurance providers serving over seven million people, about 13% of the population. Nearly half of the insured have their insurance premiums paid by their employer. Twenty per cent of 45–54 year olds have private medical insurance, the highest proportion of any age group; and 40% of people with incomes over £50,000 have private medical insurance. However, the market is stagnating due to increasing costs of premiums and improvements in the NHS.

Recent data show that there has been an increase in the number of doctors doing private work. It is estimated that 40,000 doctors across the country work for the private sector, of whom half work for private practices on a regular basis.

Tensions in NHS policy-making

Whatever organizational changes take place in the future, we can identify key tensions in NHS policy-making that are unlikely to go away but will remain key drivers in policy-making and service provision. These tensions (which overlap) can be thought of as pendulums which will be at different points in their oscillations at any one time depending on fashions and the latest media scare.

Some key tensions in NHS policy-making

Centralization	Decentralization
Centres of excellence	Local provision
National priorities	Local needs
Curing the sick	Promoting good health
Heroic measures for the individual	Greatest good for the greatest number
Accountability	Autonomy
Equity	Efficiency

Centralization/decentralization

An example of this is the increasing government control of the NHS following its major reorganization in 1974. The pendulum has swung the other way recently with the provision of Foundation Trusts and Primary Care Trusts which have much more control at local level. We are also witnessing increasing divergence in the ways health and health care are delivered in the UK, linked to the devolution of Scotland and Wales (and in due course, perhaps, Northern Ireland).

Centres of excellence/local provision

Should resources be concentrated on making a few hospitals 'regional centres' offering specialist treatments and services, and hence reducing the number of beds in local hospitals, or should community hospitals, with their ease of access for patients and relatives, be encouraged? Should women give birth in hospital or at home, and should they have the services of the same midwife throughout their pregnancy or a (more efficient) midwifery team?

National priorities/local needs

The government sets targets, but do these reflect the priorities or requirements of local communities?

Curing the sick/promoting good health

GPs bear much of the brunt of this pendulum swing. To what extent should their work become more focused on health promotion – proactive rather than reactive medicine? In the other direction are discussions about whether GPs should specialize in certain branches of medicine or be generalists who can deal appropriately with all the primary care caseload.

Heroic measures for the individual/greatest good for the greatest number

The drug Herceptin, which was licensed by the European Commission in 2006 to treat early-stage breast cancer, is likely to be cleared for clinical use in the UK too. It works on the HER2-type tumours that characterize breast cancer in 25% of breast cancer patients, about 10,000 women in the UK a year. Individual women have conducted prolonged campaigns to be prescribed the drug on the NHS. The estimated cost of Herceptin is £20,000 per patient per year, or £100 million for all the women who would need to be treated with the drug each year, one-quarter of the national budget for all cancer drugs. It is estimated that the chance of survival after three years' Herceptin treatment increases from 91.7% to 94.3%. Is the expense of the drug justified or could the money be better spent in other areas of health and health care to provide benefits for more people?

Accountability/autonomy

The Bristol Royal Infirmary case (see above) and other recent scares concerning professional practice in medicine (e.g. the Alder Hey body parts scandal, where children's body parts were removed post-mortem and kept without parental consent, and Harold Shipman, the GP who murdered many of his elderly patients) have led to demands for greater public accountability of medicine. At the moment the pendulum seems to have swung very close to full accountability, but this is a trend shared by other professions in the UK (e.g. teachers), not just the NHS. The expense of maintaining the monitoring, audit and evaluation systems (such as for the Criminal Records Bureau checks which are now obligatory for all health professionals) may lead to a swing back towards greater autonomy for health professionals.

Equity/efficiency

Equity means ensuring that services are fairly distributed so that outcomes are similar among groups. This is not the same as equal distribution of services; equity requires targeting of services to the disadvantaged and as such is seldom the most efficient (i.e. cost-effective) way of delivering services.

Case study: Problems instigating change in general practice

Originally, blood-taking (phlebotomy) was a skill exercised only by GPs; it was handed over to practice nurses in the 1960s. In 1993, a local GP decided he wanted to rationalize time and resources in his practice by relieving the practice nurses of the duty of taking blood as they were spending around 38% of their time doing phlebotomies. The GP considered that information technology had freed up the receptionists' time also. Could this relatively simple procedure not be transferred to the receptionists, thus enabling the practice nurses to spend more time on health promotion and chronic disease management programmes?

Several volunteer receptionists were sent on a one-day training course in venepuncture theory. However, there was good deal of antagonism to the idea among the practice nurses, and only one of the receptionist-phlebotomists was able to continue with her practical training. Legal and professional aspects were all addressed, and patient acceptability was assessed.

Ten years later, the scheme had been abandoned.

- What reasons can you suggest for the antagonism of the practice nurses?
- Might the receptionists also have been resistant? If so, why?
- What do you think the results of the patient acceptability study were?
- How might the GP have done better in his attempts to transform the skill mix in his general practice?

Summary

• Modern medicine has grown rapidly to become the major form of sanctioned, professional health care in the western world.

• The knowledge base of medicine is grounded in scientific principles, but there are differences of opinion within medical practice concerning the biomedical and biopsychosocial approach, the empirical approach to the individual patient and the population-based approach to decision-making advocated by EBM.

• Health professionals in the UK can be thought of as social groups and sub-groups each with its own priorities, values, history and methods of practice. Doctors share this diversity of specialities.

• Medicine is both a product of society and a reflection of it. For example, the roles of men and women see parallels in the distribution of jobs between men and women in the NHS.

• The practice of medicine varies both within and between health systems. Analysing the nature of these variations highlights how medical systems are cultural systems, and are less universal in their forms and functions than might initially be believed.

• The NHS probably offers the best value for money of any health service in the world. Its constant changes make it impossible to predict what its future shape will be, but key tensions in policy-making can be identified that will determine the parameters of what is likely to happen in the future.

Further reading

Cassell, J. (1996) The woman in the surgeon's body: understanding difference. *American Anthropologist*, **98(1)**: 41–53.

Cranney, M., Warren, E., Barton, S., Gardner, K. and Walley, T. (2001) Why do GPs not implement evidence-based guidelines? A descriptive study. *Family Practice,* **18(4)**: 359–63.

Downie, R. S. and Macnaughton, J. (2000) *Clinical Judgement: Evidence in Practice.* Oxford: Oxford University Press.

Dyer, C. (2001) Bristol inquiry condemns hospital's 'club culture'. *British Medical Journal*, **323(7306)**: 181.

Farmer, R. D. T. and Lawrenson, R. (2004) *Lecture Notes: Epidemiology and Public Health Medicine* (5th edn.). Oxford: Blackwell

Freeman, A. C. and Sweeney, K. (2001) Why general practitioners do not implement evidence: qualitative study. *British Medical Journal,* **323(7321)**: 1100–2

Lock, M. (1980) *East Asian Medicine in Urban Japan: Varieties of Medical Experience.* Berkeley, CA: University of California Press.

McManus, I. C. and Sproston, K. A. (2000) Women in hospital medicine in the United Kingdom: glass ceiling, preference, prejudice or cohort effect? *Journal of Epidemiology and Community Health*, **54**: 10–16.

Macnaughton, J. (2007) Art in hospital spaces: the role of hospitals in an aestheticized society. *International Journal of Cultural Policy* **13(1)**, 85–101.

Milne, R., Logan, R. P. H., Harwood, D., Misiewicz, J. J. and Forman, D. (1995) *Helicobacter pylori* and upper gastrointestinal disease: a survey of gastroenterologists in the United Kingdom. *Gut*, **37**: 314–18.

NHS Confederation (2006) *Why We Need Fewer Hospital Beds.* Report available at http://www.nhsconfed.org.

Ohnuki-Tierney, E. (1984) *Illness and Culture in Contemporary Japan: an Anthropological View.* Cambridge: Cambridge University Press.

Payer, L. (1990) *Medicine and Culture: Notions of Health and Sickness.* London: Gollancz.

Chapter 5

Health and health care in the folk sector: complementary and alternative medicine

Introduction

The folk sector is made up of all the health and healing resources other than those of the professional and popular sectors of a particular society in a given period. While the terminology may vary, an all-embracing term used to describe the sector in the West is 'complementary and alternative medicine' (CAM). In many other societies CAM is referred to as 'traditional medicine'. The boundaries within and between CAM and the professional sector are not always sharp or fixed. Many kinds of CAM are becoming increasingly professionalized and it is possible to obtain different 'folk' treatments through the NHS. It is also often hard to distinguish between CAM and the popular sector, but one clear difference is that payment is normally made for services in the CAM sector whereas interventions in the popular sector are usually free. CAM in the UK has traditionally been seen by most people as the last step in the hierarchy of resort. However, it is now increasingly being used at any stage of health-seeking behaviour.

The folk sector encompasses a vast array of forms, beliefs and practices, and, like the other two sectors, it is rapidly changing. On the whole,

Lecture Notes: *The Social Basis of Medicine*, 1st edition. By Andrew Russell. Published 2009 by Blackwell Publishing. ISBN: 978-1-4051-3912-0

it is not as well organized as the professional sector is in the UK, but it is more clearly defined than the popular sector.

This chapter covers the following topics
What is CAM?
Why is it important to know about CAM?
Forms of CAM
Why might CAM work?
The integration of CAM into health systems worldwide

What is CAM?

The labels given to practices in the folk sector are either based on their relationship to the professional sector (the first four in the bullet list below) or are descriptive terms in their own right.

What's in a name?

The folk sector is known by different labels in the UK. None of these is value-neutral:
- Complementary.
- Alternative.
- Non-orthodox.
- Non-conventional.
- Holistic, natural, harmless.
- Unregulated, non-statutory.
- Unproved, irrational, unscientific.

Comments on CAM terms

Complementary vs. alternative

Complementary and alternative are used synonymously but imply different things about the relationship of the folk sector to the professional sector:

- Complementary suggests the professional sector is primary, whereas the folk sector is a subsidiary but integrated part of the system.
- Alternative suggests a much more oppositional relationship – i.e. 'instead of' the professional sector.

'Non-orthodox' and 'non-conventional'

These suggest something non-conformist or contravening agreed standards of practice about CAM:

- Some people use forms of CAM as their mainstream, 'orthodox' medicine.
- Some kinds of CAM are extremely conformist within the parameters of what they do.

'Holistic', 'natural' and 'harmless'

These reflect positive views of CAM, but ones which are not altogether accurate and may be misleading:

- 'Holistic' – not all types of CAM are 'holistic' in their approach; some forms of treatment are quite narrow in their focus. Conversely, the 'biopsychosocial' model of medicine is intrinsically holistic.
- 'Natural' – one of the most misused words in the English language?
  - It echoes a romantic view in which nature is a synonym for goodness. As such it is often used by advertisers to promote products in a misleading way.
  - Much good (professional) medical practice is also 'natural' (e.g. treatment with aspirin, the active ingredient salicylic acid derived from willow bark).
  - Many of the practices of CAM, it could be argued, are invasive and 'unnatural' (e.g. acupuncture).
- 'Harmless' – deadly nightshade is an example of an attractive, 'natural' product which would be disastrous if used as a herbal remedy because it is toxic!

'Unregulated' and 'non-statutory'

- An increasing number of branches of CAM, such as chiropractic and osteopathy, are well regulated (i.e. controlled by state legislation) – a growing trend in complementary therapies in general.
- All complementary medicine delivered by conventional health professionals is covered by their statutory frameworks and agreements.

'Unproved', 'irrational' and 'unscientific'

- Unproved – there are also growing bodies of evidence, including some randomized controlled trials, which have 'proved' some types of CAM to be effective. The majority of practices in western biomedicine are not 'proved' in this way either (see Chapter 4).
- 'Irrational' – while some kinds of CAM may at first sight seem 'irrational', research is now explaining some of what were previously mysteries surrounding the apparent efficacy of certain treatments such as acupuncture or hypnosis.
- Many forms of CAM are based on long and complex traditions which 'make sense' in their own terms.
- 'Unscientific' – yet it is being covered (and in some cases particular techniques and approaches taught) in increasing numbers of medical schools in the UK.

So what is CAM? This definition used by the Cochrane Collaboration is widely accepted. It settles on the fact that CAM is essentially anything other than the dominant health system of a society at a particular time:

'A broad domain of healing resources that encompasses all health systems, modalities, and practices and their accompanying theories and beliefs, other than those intrinsic to the politically dominant health system of a particular society or culture in a given historical period . . . Boundaries within CAM and between the CAM domain and that of the dominant system are not always sharp or fixed.'

CAM is certainly not a minor part of health care. There are currently 50,000 registered complementary practitioners in the UK compared with 30,000

GPs. However, if doctors are to give advice or make recommendations about CAM to a patient, it is important that they have confidence in the practitioner (if not the method). The British Register of Complementary Medicine (ICM-BRCP) maintains a register of CAM practitioners who have proved their competence, either by completing an approved course or by being assessed by the Registration Panel. They also agree to abide by a Code of Ethics and Practice and have full practitioner insurance. Individual forms of CAM also have their own registration boards.

Why is it important to know about CAM?

- The changing attitude of the British Medical Association (BMA).
- Training requirements set by the General Medical Council (GMC).
- Doctors' attitudes to and use of CAM.
- Medical students' attitudes to and use of CAM.
- Public use of CAM.
- International comparisons.

The changing attitude of the BMA

There has been a marked change in attitude to CAM by the BMA in recent years. In a report published in 1986, for example, the BMA stated:

'About the only aspect of these therapies which is common to all is that they are not based on orthodox scientific principles . . .

. . . The fact is that the steadily developing body of orthodox medical knowledge has led to large, demonstrable, and reproducible benefits for mankind, of a scale which cannot be matched by alternative approaches.'

By 1993, this attitude had softened, as witnessed by the statement:

'It is clear that there are many encouraging initiatives currently taking place in the field of non-conventional therapy, and it is to be hoped that good practice can be extrapolated for general use.'

Training requirements set by the GMC

The GMC's report 'Tomorrow's Doctors' lists the requirements that graduates in medicine in the UK must be able to show they can meet. Among them graduates should be aware of the following:

- Many patients are interested in and choose to use a wide range of alternative and complementary therapies.
- The existence and range of such therapies.
- Why some patients use them.
- How these might affect other types of treatment that patients are receiving.

Doctors' attitudes to and use of CAM

The approach of many doctors to CAM, like that of their professional organization the BMA, is changing. While there is considerable variation among surveys, nearly half the doctors practising in the UK think that CAM is either useful or effective. Younger doctors tend to be more positive about it than older doctors. Ten per cent of GPs are actively involved in practising it, while more than a third of GP partnerships provide access to CAM for their NHS patients.

Medical students' attitudes to and use of CAM

Medical students' approach to CAM is also changing. Surveys indicate that over two-thirds of medical students (more women than men) now believe CAM offers effective treatments, and at least a third know someone who has used it. Twenty per cent of medical students have used CAM themselves, but often feel they don't know enough about individual therapies to feel confident in referring patients to them.

Public use of CAM

Recent studies in the UK have shown:

- Approximately 33% of people have used CAM at some time; 11% have used it in past year.

- More women than men use CAM (this is also true of conventional health care).
- Highest use rates are among 35–60 year olds.
- Highest use rates are found among the higher socio-economic groups and education levels.
- It is used more in the South than the North.
- Use is often linked to more chronic and difficult-to-manage diseases.
- It is frequently used in combination with orthodox medicine (i.e. is complementary to it).
- People using CAM are unlikely to inform their NHS GP.

International comparisons

Figure 5.1 is based on WHO data, but has to be treated with caution. We cannot be certain that the studies from which these figures derive were comparing like with like. What kinds of CAM are included? When were the studies conducted? The UK figure, for example, is based on lifetime use of eight named therapies. A study in the US in 2002, for example, indicated that 36% of people had used CAM. But this was after 'prayer for health' and 'megavitamin use' were excluded; if they are included, the figure rises to 62%. We do not know whether these categories of CAM were included in the WHO studies. Age differences between populations will obviously also have an effect on the likelihood of people having used CAM 'in their lifetime'. Despite these issues, it appears that CAM is even more widely used in some other developed countries than it is in the UK.

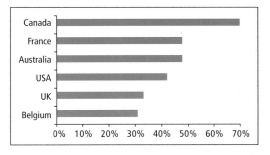

Figure 5.1 Percentage of the population who have used CAM at least once, selected developed countries (Source: WHO 2002).

Forms of CAM

The diversity of forms of CAM makes categorizing them difficult. Often individual practitioners will deliver more than one form of CAM, and there can be considerable variation within and between practitioners.

Biologically-based practices make use of substances found in nature such as herbs, diets and vitamins, outside any normal doses prescribed by conventional medicine. Examples of such practices include herbal medicine, naturopathy and aromatherapy.

Some forms of CAM make use of *energy fields* which are believed to surround and penetrate the human body. These fields may or may not be verifiable according to the canons of western science. Examples include acupuncture, reflexology and Reiki healing.

Manipulative and body-based practices depend on manipulation or the movement of one or more body parts for their effects. Examples include chiropractic, osteopathy, shiatsu and the Alexander technique.

Some practices are designed to enhance the *mind*'s ability to affect *bodily* functions and symptoms. Examples include hypnotherapy, visualization, relaxation and spiritual healing. Other practices may be more purely psychological in their approach or effects, such as shamanic healing and counselling.

Other forms of CAM offer *complete systems* of theory and practice which have evolved apart from (and sometimes earlier than) conventional medicine. Examples are homoeopathy, Ayurveda and Unani (the latter two the traditional therapies of South Asia and the Arab world respectively).

There is a significant degree of overlap within and between therapies. For example, shiatsu massage involves the practitioner applying varying rhythmic pressure with the fingers on parts of the body that are believed to be important for the flow of a vital energy called *qi*. Hence shiatsu could be included in either the 'massage' or 'energy fields' category.

We deal below with what are probably the six most popular forms of CAM practised in the UK.

Questions to ask of any form of CAM therapy

1 What is the background to your therapy (i.e. its history)?
2 What are its fundamental concepts?
3 What diagnosis and treatment does it do?
4 What research has there been into the therapy?
5 Does it work?
6 Is it safe?
7 What are the risks and benefits of this therapy?
8 Would you refer a patient of yours to it?
9 Would you use it?

Herbal medicine

Herbal medicine uses plants for healing purposes, a tradition that pre-dates modern medical practice. Indeed, herbalism is what much modern medical practice is based on.

Examples of pharmaceutical products derived from plants

Aspirin – willow bark
Digoxin – foxglove
Quinine – cinchona bark
Morphine – opium poppy
Herbal medicine is different from conventional pharmacology in several key aspects

Use of whole plants – rather than isolating the 'active ingredient' of a plant product, herbal practitioners tend to use unpurified, whole-plant products, which are seen as working together synergistically. Toxicity may also be reduced when the whole plant is used rather than its active ingredients only, a feature known as 'buffering'.
Combining herbs – a variety of herbs may be selected and used in combination according to the characteristics of the individual patient and skill of the herbalist. The principles of synergy and buffering may apply equally to plants in combination.

Diagnosis – can be very different compared to conventional medicine. Chronic fatigue syndrome, for example, a difficult and ambiguous diagnosis to make in western medicine, may be described, according to the patient's individual characteristics, in Chinese herbal medicine as 'the retention of dampness (with some damp-heat) with deficiency of *qi* (spleen, lung, kidney) and depletion of yin'.

Chinese traditional medicine makes much use of herbs, with an underlying philosophy that there are two complementary properties – yin and yang – and that herbs are either 'cooling' (yin) or 'stimulating' (yang). The idea of a life force (*qi*) which may be blocked is also a feature of Chinese traditional medicine, which makes it a type of energy medicine also.

Homoeopathy

Homoeopathy is an example of a complete system of medical theory and practice. It was founded by Samuel Hahnemann (1755–1843), a German physician who lived in Dresden. It is based on the principle that like cures like, i.e. that the presenting symptoms can be exacerbated by a herb, animal product or mineral and hence stimulate the body's 'vital force' into restoring health. (In this it contrasts with allopathic medicine.) This is done using very low-dose preparations. These are created by a process of serial dilution and succussion (vigorous shaking). The minimum dose is said to be that which releases the curative power of the product while removing contraindications. However, the greater the number of times this process is repeated, the more potent the remedy is considered to be, although many homoeopathic medicines are diluted to such a degree that nothing material exists beyond the fifth dilution (the law of infinitesimals).

One of the first homoeopathic doctors to practise in England was Frederick Foster Hervey Quin. In 1820 he travelled to Italy, working as a physician in Naples and Rome, before taking up homoeopathy in 1826. He returned to England as physician to Prince Leopold of Saxe-Coburg (widower of George IV's daughter, Charlotte) and set up the first homoeopathic practice in London in 1832. He founded the British Homeopathic Society in 1844 and the London Homoeopathic Hospital (LHH) in 1850. During a cholera outbreak in 1854, the mortality rate in allopathic hospitals was 51.8%, while in the LHH it was 16.4%. The support for homoeopathy among the aristocracy during the nineteenth century meant it nearly became the officially sanctioned medical system in the UK. There are still five NHS homoeopathic hospitals in the UK.

Osteopathy/Chiropractic

Osteopathy and chiropractic are two distinct but related types of manipulative therapy. Osteopathy was founded by Andrew Taylor Still in the US in the nineteenth century. In addition to manipulation of the spine, it assumes that impaired blood supply causes illness. Chiropractic, established by another American, Daniel David Palmer, assumes that the nerves that control posture and movement can become inflamed and cause referred pain. During the twentieth century, the range of ailments for which osteopathy and chiropractic were regarded as beneficial (among both practitioners themselves and the wider medical profession) narrowed so that now musculoskeletal disorders are the main focus.

Problems which the British Osteopathic Association lists as being relievable by osteopathy are:
- Back pain.
- Arthritic pain.
- Menstrual pain.
- Repetitive strain injury.
- Shoulder and neck pain, including frozen shoulder.
- Sleeping difficulties.
- Neuralgia and sinus pain.
- Teeth grinding.
- Irritable bowel syndrome.
- Sciatica.
- Mobility problems.
- Sports injury.

- Postural problems caused by pregnancy, driving or work strain.
- Joint pain, muscular aches, pains and strains.
- 'Tennis elbow' (lateral epicondylitis).
- Asthma and other respiratory problems.
- Colic and sleeplessness in babies.

Chiropractors usually also include headache and migraine as amenable to treatment by their form of medicine.

The titles 'chiropractor' and 'osteopath' are protected by law in the UK and, since 1998 for osteopathy and 2001 for chiropractic, it has been a criminal offence to describe oneself as any sort of chiropractor or osteopath without being registered with the General Chiropractic Council or General Osteopathic Council respectively.

Acupuncture

Acupuncture originated in China at least 2000 years ago. It is based on a theory of 12 interconnected energy channels (meridians) which link all the internal organs and body systems in an organic whole. By inserting fine needles in the acupuncture points along these meridians and stimulating them in specific ways the entire body can be controlled and regulated. Acupuncture points are said to be marked by higher electrical conductance than the surrounding skin and hence are places where the flow of energy (*qi*) can be most easily influenced. It is important that the needles are inserted in the correct directions for the effects they are supposed to have. The British Acupuncture Council insists that members use single-use, pre-sterilized disposable needles. Other organizations in the UK such as the British Medical Acupuncture Society and the British Academy of Western Medical Acupuncture cater for conventional health professionals who practise acupuncture.

Naturopathy

Naturopathy uses combination of dietary change and other interventions to effect change using 'natural' methods that assist the body's own ability to recover from illness and injury. Naturopathy tends to be holistic in approach and may involve a broad range of other therapies, including manipulative therapies, hydrotherapy, herbalism, acupuncture and counselling. The seven principles of naturopathy are:

1 Do no harm.
2 Nature has healing power.
3 Identify and treat the cause.
4 Treat the whole person.
5 The naturopath is a teacher.
6 Prevention is the best cure.
7 Establish health and well-being.

Naturopathy in the UK is closely allied with osteopathy and naturopaths registered with the General Council and Register of Naturopaths will have completed either a three- or four-year full-time degree level course, or a two-year postgraduate Naturopathic Diploma (ND). ND practitioners do not perform minor surgery or have prescribing rights.

Why might CAM work?

- Specific therapeutic effect
- Quality of interaction
- Placebo effect
- Natural history of disease
- How do we evaluate effectiveness anyway?

In order to be able to say that a particular CAM treatment has 'worked', we would have to be able to say it posed no risk to the patient and was of some benefit. This benefit can be direct (i.e. specific to the treatment itself) or indirect (i.e. dependent on the context of treatment – the same context could be efficacious irrespective of the treatment). Randomized controlled trials are one way of distinguishing them, but there are difficulties (see below). However, even if no specific therapeutic effect can be demonstrated, a treatment may still 'work' if it gives the patient benefit of some kind and causes no harm.

Specific therapeutic effect

Some products and practices have a specific therapeutic effect – that is, a pharmacological or other effect that is independent of the context in which they are administered. For example, the herbal medicine St John's Wort (*Hypericum perforatum*) has been proved in randomized controlled trials to be effective in the treatment of mild to moderate depression, with fewer side-effects than pharmaceutical antidepressants such as amitriptyline.

Where a specific therapeutic effect can be demonstrated, then the possibility of specific adverse effects must also be considered. In the case of herbalism, for example, toxicity and possible interactions with other treatments must be considered. St John's Wort, for example, is contraindicated in cases where anti-retroviral drugs (prescribed for example for HIV) are being taken, since one of the active ingredients in the herb lowers the effectiveness of the anti-retroviral. Similarly, the herb interacts with the oral contraceptive pill, leading to reduced levels in the blood, breakthrough bleeding and the risk of unwanted pregnancy. Given that patients are unlikely to tell their doctor that they are taking a CAM product (see above) it is important to be aware of these contraindications and inform patients of them.

Quality of interaction

Even where no specific effect can be proved, a therapy may 'work' simply because the patient enjoys a high-quality interaction with the practitioner. Studies have shown that appointments with a CAM practitioner (of any sort) almost always last longer than appointments in most NHS practices.

Many patients are dissatisfied with conventional medicine, both because of its time constraints and because of what is seen as its overly biological focus. The holistic approach of many forms of CAM, with its detailed questions about medical history, diet, lifestyle, sleeping patterns, relationships, likes and dislikes, is gratifying. While the therapist builds up a 'whole' picture, many patients find it therapeutic to have the opportunity to talk at length about themselves. Even if no 'cure' is effected, their sense of well-being may be enhanced – they 'feel better'.

Placebo effect

A placebo is an inert substance having no discernible pharmacological effect. The placebo effect is harnessed whenever a product is administered that either has no active ingredient or one that is not known to affect the condition being treated in any way. In randomized controlled trials the placebo effect can be observed in up to 50% of cases. Procedures as well as products can have a placebo effect. The efficacy of many forms of CAM is attributable to the placebo effect – that is, the context of the treatment is therapeutic rather than the treatment itself. There are three forms of context effect:

1 Treatment characteristics (e.g. colour, size, shape of drug).

2 Practitioner characteristics (e.g. reputation, setting, displayed competence).

3 Patient characteristics (e.g. perception of staff, trust, past experience of treatment working, beliefs).

Natural history of disease

It is estimated that up to 90% of acute diseases are 'self-limiting' – the patient will get better regardless of the treatment given. If a treatment is given, though, and the patient subsequently gets better, people will often attribute this to the treatment rather than to the natural history of their disease.

How do we measure effectiveness anyway?

- Methodological difficulties
- Infrastructural difficulties
- Safety
- Access?
- Value for money?

Methodological difficulties

Non-standardized treatments

Many kinds of CAM offer individualized treatment so it can be hard to identify what aspect of a particular treatment is significant. What about the role of the therapeutic relationship itself? This could have at least a placebo effect on outcomes. Complementary therapists tend to speak a different language from medical science. How can you measure something as subtle as *qi*, for example – assuming that doctors accept it might exist in the first place?

Running a study

It can be hard to recruit patients to a study and insufficient patient numbers may be a problem. Where someone is paying for treatment, they may not wish to take part in a study where they risk being a 'control' who receives the placebo. Even where they are willing to take part, it can be hard to 'blind' patients to their treatment allocation. How can you fake a massage, for example, and can you expect a highly skilled acupuncturist to deliberately insert needles in the 'wrong' place?

Intra-disciplinary variation (e.g. in acupuncture)

Many forms of CAM demonstrate considerable variation between different branches or indeed among individual practitioners. Such intra-disciplinary variation can mask the effect of particular forms of treatment.

Infrastructural difficulties

Lack of funding

Properly run trials can be expensive and are usually carried out by hospitals, universities or pharmaceutical companies. Among these organizations, research into unconventional therapies may have little appeal. Most herbal remedies, for instance, have been in use for centuries and there is no incentive to go for financially attractive patents.

Lack of academic infrastructure/research skills

Partly because of the difficulties of funding appropriate trials, and partly because of the lack of academic input into researching CAM, there is a general lack of academic infrastructure and research skills.

Safety

Safety (or absence of risk) is a weaker requirement than proof of benefit. There are a number of safety requirements that any CAM practitioner should fulfil:

- Practise only within competence.

- Take sufficient medical history to ensure no contraindications.
- Do not advise changes to conventional treatment without consulting doctor.
- (Ideally) communicate with doctor over diagnosis, treatment, duration.
- Have current registration and follow codes of conduct.
- Hold full insurance.
- Be able to supply full references.

Another risk that should be acknowledged is the danger of individuals receiving CAM treatment deciding to dispense with their biomedical treatment altogether. This may be serious in the case of unproven CAM therapies for life-threatening diseases such as cancer.

The integration of CAM in other health systems

New developments for CAM in the UK

The Complementary and Natural Healthcare Council (CNHC)

The CNHC is a regulatory body set up in April 2008, funded by the Department of Health and modelled on the General Medical Council (see Chapter 4). It gives practitioners of the therapies it covers the opportunity to register (though they are not obliged to do so). Registration indicates that the practitioner has met certain entry requirements (i.e. has a recognized qualification) and subscribes to a set of professional standards. Breach of these standards may mean that the practitioner is referred for 'fitness to practise' procedures, which could result in their removal from the register. All the CNHC's council members are lay people appointed through an independent process. These people are not part of the professional bodies representing the complementary therapies in question.

The following therapies are involved in the CNHC:

Alexander technique.
Bowen technique.
Cranial therapy.
Homoeopathy.
Massage therapy.
Naturopathy.
Nutritional therapy.
Shiatsu.
Yoga therapy.

In addition, aromatherapists, reflexologists and Reiki practitioners will also become eligible to join the register.

The government is to consider whether to establish statutory regulation of acupuncture, herbal medicine and traditional Chinese medicine. These three therapies have been chosen because they involve more invasive procedures (skin piercing) and the ingestion of herbal substances, and therefore may pose greater potential dangers than other, less invasive therapies.

Traditional medicine – CAM in other parts of the world

In other parts of the world, what in the UK is a CAM therapy may be regarded as the traditional medicine (TM) of the area. The World Health Organization (WHO) in particular has expressed enthusiasm for incorporating traditional medicine into the official health systems of developing countries. It is seen as offering an accessible and affordable alternative to allopathic, western medicine for people living in rural areas. In some parts of the developed world, such as Taiwan and Japan, 'traditional' medicine coexists with more conventional medicine.

Aims of the WHO's Traditional Medicine Strategy 2002–5

- Integrate TM/CAM into national health care systems.
- Promote safety, efficacy and quality of TM/CAM.
- Increase availability and affordability of TM/CAM.
- Promote therapeutically sound use of TM/CAM.

Two policy models exist for the integration of TM into medical practice. The *integrated approach*, as practised in China and Vietnam, aims to teach both forms of medicine and to enable both to be practised, by the same practitioner if possible. The *parallel approach* is somewhat less ambitious and aims at separate development within a national health system. Examples of this are found in India and South Korea, although in the case of some colleges in India students take a foundation year that is common to both Ayurveda and conventional medicine.

Summary

- Complementary and alternative medicines are part of the folk sector.
- The BMA has become more favourable towards CAM in recent years.
- Doctors need to know about CAM in order to understand what their patients may be taking alongside conventional medicine and treatments.
- The six most common forms of CAM in the UK are herbal medicine, chiropractic, osteopathy, acupuncture, homoeopathy and naturopathy.
- There are various reasons why CAM might work; only one of these has to do with the specific therapeutic properties of the treatment.
- The Complementary and Natural Healthcare Council (CNHC) is a government-appointed body set up to regulate the activities of a number of CAM therapies in the UK.
- In other parts of the world, what in the UK is CAM is regarded as traditional medicine and coexists either in parallel or integrated with orthodox western medicine.

Further reading

Barry, C. (2006) The role of evidence in alternative medicine: contrasting biomedical and anthropological approaches. *Social Science and Medicine*, 62: 2646–57.

Bodeker, G. (2001) Lessons on integration from the developing world's experience. *British Medical Journal*, 322: 164–7 (Part of a themed issue: Integrated medicine: orthodox meets alternative).

Fulder, S. (1997) *The Handbook of Alternative and Complementary Medicine: the Essential Health Companion.* London: Vermilion.

Furnham, A., Hanna, D. and Vincent, A. (1995) Medical students' attitudes to complementary medical therapies. *Complementary Therapies in Medicine*, 3(4): 212–19

Owen, D. K., Lewith, G. and Stephens, C. R. (2001) Can doctors respond to patients' increasing interest in complementary and alternative medicine? *British Medical Journal*, 322: 154–7.

Saks, M. (2003) *Orthodox and Alternative Medicine: Politics, Professionalization and Health Care.* London: Sage.

Szegedi, A., Kohnen, R., Dienel, A., and Kieser, M. (2005) Acute treatment of moderate to severe depression with hypericum extract WS 5570 (St John's Wort): randomised controlled double blind non-inferiority trial versus paroxetine. *British Medical Journal*, **330**: 503.

World Health Organization (2002) *WHO Traditional Medicine Strategy 2002–5*. http://whqlibdoc.who.int/hq/2002/WHO_EDM_TRM_2002.1.pdf.

Zollman, C. and Vickers, A. J. (2000) *ABC of Complementary Medicine*. London: BMJ *Books*. (Also available as separate chapters online in various 1999 issues of the *British Medical Journal*, 319.)

Chapter 6

The consultation

Introduction

Everyday in the UK about one million people consult their GP. In any two-week period, approximately 10% of adults and children are likely to see their GP, a proportion which has changed very little over the past 30 years. Girls and women have an average of five NHS GP consultations a year, while boys and men have four. The likelihood of visiting a GP increases with age. According to the General Household Survey, 12% of adults aged 16–24 are likely to consult their GP in a 13-day period, compared to over 20% amongst those aged 75 and over.

Often, and increasingly so with the reduction in numbers of 'single-handed' general practices where continuity of care is more likely, the two people who meet in such a consultation are complete strangers prior to the event. Yet, within minutes, patients are likely to be revealing some of the most intimate details of their physical and/ or emotional states. They may be asked to remove their clothing for examination. In other words, the patient is giving control to the authority of the GP to an extent which, in a different context,

would be extraordinary. There is little parity in such an exchange – it would be regarded as extremely unprofessional for the doctor to disclose any of their own personal problems or to undress, for example. What the doctor is expected to provide in return is honesty, integrity, the keeping of secrets, accurate recording and respect.

The behaviour we observe between doctors and patients in a consultation is only acceptable because it is structured and follows a socially agreed pattern. Yet within these parameters the manner of the interaction can vary considerably. Different types of doctor–patient interaction can be recognized. Social factors such as class, age and ethnicity impinge on the consultation to affect what takes place and the outcome. New technologies promise to push the model of the doctor–patient encounter in new and previously unimagined directions.

Lecture Notes: *The Social Basis of Medicine*, 1st edition. By Andrew Russell. Published 2009 by Blackwell Publishing. ISBN: 978-1-4051-3912-0

This chapter covers the following topics

The roles and goals of doctors and patients
The anatomy of the consultation
Types of doctor–patient relationship
Doctor–patient relationships in practice
The benefits of patient-centred medicine
New technologies and the doctor–patient encounter

The roles and goals of doctors and patients

The doctor–patient relationship contains certain expectations about ways of behaving that are generally held by all members of society. These provide structure and coherence to what happens in the clinical encounter. A doctor behaving in the manner depicted in Figure 6.1, for example, would lack credibility and trust in the eyes of the patient.

The people involved in the clinical encounter play different roles depending on their position – doctor, patient, other carers, etc. Roles are social positions which carry privileges, obligations, rights and expectations for the bearer. Depending on the nature of the relationship some roles, such as the doctor's, can be more active, while others (such as the patient's) can be more passive. The doctor may assume a position of authority over the patient and their other carers, and patients and carers are generally willing to grant this authority (Table 6.1). They are, after all, looking for the doctor's knowledge and his or her capacity to access the health services on their behalf.

In order to gain the privileges of the sick role, however, patients are expected to fulfil certain obligations. There is an expectation that they will engage in health-seeking behaviour that will

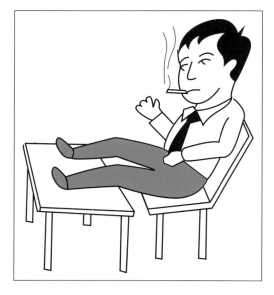

Figure 6.1 The bad doctor.

enable them to get better (in the case of acute illness) or sustain themselves (in the case of chronic illness), and that they will seek some kind of professional help, if they can, to do this.

Doctors also have obligations to fulfil. These are enshrined in codes of practice such as the GMC's 'Good Medical Practice'.

'Good Medical Practice' (2006)

The duties of a doctor registered with the General Medical Council

Patients must be able to trust doctors with their lives and health. To justify that trust you must show respect for human life and you must:
- Make the care of your patient your first concern.
- Protect and promote the health of patients and the public.
- Provide a good standard of practice and care:
  ○ keep your professional knowledge and skills up to date;
  ○ recognize and work within the limits of your competence;
  ○ work with colleagues in the ways that best serve patients' interests.
- Treat patients as individuals and respect their dignity:
  ○ treat patients politely and considerately;
  ○ respect patients' right to confidentiality.
- Work in partnership with patients:
  ○ listen to patients and respond to their concerns and preferences;
  ○ give patients the information they want or need in a way they can understand;

> ○ respect patients' right to reach decisions with you about their treatment and care;
> ○ support patients in caring for themselves to improve and maintain their health.
> • Be honest and open and act with integrity:
> ○ act without delay if you have good reason to believe that you or a colleague may be putting patients at risk;
> ○ never discriminate unfairly against patients or colleagues;
> ○ never abuse your patients' trust in you, or the public's trust in the profession;
> ○ you are personally accountable for your professional practice and must always be prepared to justify your decisions and actions.

These are the obligations to which every doctor in the UK is expected to adhere. They have changed subtly over the years to reflect the changing nature of the doctor–patient relationship and the need to emphasize actions rather than words (e.g. the phrase 'work in partnership with patients' used to be 'respect the right of patients to be fully involved in decisions about their care').

Questioning roles

Roles are not 'cut and dried'. Circumstances such as the following affect whether or not a role is adopted, its components and how it is performed:
• Trivial illness (e.g. a cold) may not warrant adoption of sick role.
• Chronic illness can be such that a person adopts the sick role only when their illness is worse than usual (see Chapter 12).
• Severity of the illness determines the number and nature of activities a person will give up when adopting the sick role.
• Some may adopt the sick role even though nothing objectively can be found to indicate they are ill (4–9% of general practice patients are estimated to suffer from hypochondriasis, a fear that signs and symptoms are indicative of a serious illness despite medical reassurance that they are not).
• Malingerers will continue with the sick role even when they are technically better. People on the upward trajectory to health are called convalescents.
• Conflicting roles may occur when there is a shortage of resources and the doctor has to act in ways that do not maximally benefit a patient.
• There are different styles within the 'doctor role' which are partly dependent on circumstances and culture. The style adopted in an Accident and Emergency Department, for example, is likely to be different from the style adopted in a palliative care facility. The way a doctor behaves in Tashkent (Uzbekistan), say, is likely to be different from how a doctor behaves in Tottenham (UK).
• There are different styles within the 'patient role' which are partly dependent on circumstances and culture.

Table 6.1 The role of doctor and patient.

Patient = Sick role (passive)	Privileges	Exempt from normal duties
		Regarded as in need of care
		Not seen as responsible for own state
	Obligations	Get well as soon as possible
		Seek professional help
Doctor = Professional role (active)	Expectations and obligations	Apply skill to benefit of patient/community
		High degree of professionalism
		Objective, dispassionate
	Rights	Examine patients physically
		Ask intimate questions

Cultural diversity in illness expression

The expression of illness, the way in which an individual performs the patient role, differs markedly both within and across cultures. Suffering and discomfort are signalled in ways that are learned; they are not innate. Here are extracts from transcripts of two patients living in Boston, MA, describing the symptoms of eye problems, long-sightedness in the case of patients A and B, and short-sightedness in the case of patients C and D.

Interviewer	Patient A	Patient B
'What seems to be the trouble?'	'I can't see to thread a needle or read a paper'	'I have a constant headache and my eyes seem to get all red and burny'
'Anything else?'	'No, I can't recall any'	'No, just that it lasts all day long and I even wake up with it sometimes'

Interviewer	Patient C	Patient D
'What seems to be the trouble?'	'I can't see across the street'	'My eyes seem very burny, especially the right eye . . . Two or three months ago I woke with my eye swollen. I bathed it and it did go away but there was still the burny sensation'
'Anything else?'	'I had been experiencing headaches, but it may be that I'm early in the menopause'	'Yes, there always seems to be a red spot beneath this eye . . .'
'Anything else?'	'No'	'Well, my eyes feel very heavy . . . at night they bother me most'
		(source: Zola 1973)

These transcripts provide very different accounts of similar problems. Patients A and C give accounts based on function (what they can't see) and tend to explain away symptoms ('it may be that I'm early in the menopause') and stop the dialogue quickly. Patients B and D, by contrast, give accounts based on symptomatology and feelings, and use quite florid language.

Patients A and C come from the Irish-American community; Patients B and D are from the Italian-American community.

In many cultures, it is more common to express emotional problems through recourse to physical symptoms than by using abstract, psychological terms. This is known as *somatization* and can often be misinterpreted by doctors from a different cultural background as indicating the presence of a physical disease. Often symptoms expressed are vague and generalized (e.g. feeling tired, weak or having 'pains everywhere'). In some cultures, more specific physical symptoms may be invoked, such as headaches, palpitations, weight loss and dizziness. Particular organs may become the focus of anxiety: in China, the liver, spleen, kidney or heart; in Iran and Punjab, the heart. In the UK and other parts of the Anglophone world, the bowels are a particularly important focus of concern. The expression of physical complaints in these organs is often a metaphorical and more socially acceptable way of indicating emotional distress.

Explanatory models: establishing convergent goals

Explanatory models (EMs) are a useful way of thinking about and explaining the different notions about a particular illness episode and how it should be treated which are brought to the clinical encounter by patients and their lay and/or professional carers. They are derived from the knowledge base (theoretical and experiential) and cultural background of the individuals concerned. EMs explain some or all of the following:

- Cause of ill health.
- Symptoms and their timing.
- The bodily processes generating the symptoms.
- The course and severity of the ill health.
- Appropriate treatment.

EMs, particularly patients' EMs, are fluid and can be edited and change over time. Patients' EMs also tend to be fragmented, multifaceted and embedded in their social context. In comparison, a doctor's EM is rooted in biomedical understanding and its scientific context. The goal of an effective consultation is that the EMs of all groups, which may be very different and even conflicting, should converge. However, the power dynamics and structural limitations of the consultation (e.g. time-limited GP appointments)

mean that often the patient's EM is not properly expressed.

The anatomy of the consultation

The Calgary-Cambridge framework for communication describes in detail the many facets of competent clinical communication. It presents an exhaustive list of procedures, not all of which would be required in any one interaction. The list illustrates the wide range of abilities which the physician needs to have at his or her disposal. Often these are called 'skills', but this runs the risk of making them sound like a matter of technique or style: rather, they should be part of humane practice, and it should always be remembered that what is said is as important as how it is said. The practice of good communication needs continuous development throughout one's medical career.

The Calgary-Cambridge Framework for Communication

Initiating the session

Establishing initial rapport
  1 Greets patient and obtains patient's name.
  2 Introduces self and clarifies role.
  3 Demonstrates interest and respect, attends to patient's physical comfort.

Identifying the reason(s) for the consultation
  4 The opening question: identifies the problems or issues that the patient wishes to address ('What would you like to discuss today?').
  5 Listening to the patient's opening statement: listens attentively without interrupting or directing patient's response.
  6 Screening: checks and confirms list of problems (e.g. 'So that's headaches and tiredness. Is there anything else you'd like to discuss today?').
  7 Agenda-setting: negotiates agenda, taking both patient's and physician's needs into account.

Gathering information

Exploration of problems
  8 Patient's narrative: encourages patient to tell the story of the problem(s) in own words, from when they first started to the present (clarifying reason for presenting now).
  9 Question style: uses open and closed questioning techniques, moving appropriately from open-ended to closed.
  10 Listening: listens attentively, allowing patient to complete statements without interruption and leaving space for patient to think before answering or go on after pausing.
  11 Facilitate response: facilitate patient's responses verbally and non-verbally (e.g. use of encouragement, silence, repetition, paraphrasing, interpreting).

(continued on p. 72)

(continued)

12 Clarification: checks out statements which are vague or need amplification (e.g. 'Could you explain what you mean by light-headed?').

13 Internal summary: periodically summarizes to verify own understanding of what the patient has said; invites patient to correct interpretation or provide further information.

14 Language: uses concise, easily understood questions and comments, avoids or adequately explains jargon.

Understanding the patient's perspective

15 Ideas and concerns: determines and acknowledges patient's ideas (beliefs about cause) and concerns (worries) regarding each problem.

16 Effects: determines how each problem affects the patient's life.

17 Expectations: determines patient's goals (the help the patient had expected for each problem).

18 Feelings and thoughts: encourages expression of the patient's feelings and thoughts.

19 Cues: picks up verbal and non-verbal cues (body language, speech, facial expression, affect); checks and acknowledges as appropriate.

Providing structure to the consultation

20 Internal summary: summarizes at the end of a specific line of inquiry to confirm understanding before moving on to the next section.

21 Signposting: progresses from one section to another using transitional statements; includes rationale for next section.

22 Sequencing: structures interview in logical sequence.

23 Timing: attends to timing and keeps interview on task.

Building the relationship

Developing rapport

24 Non-verbal behaviour: demonstrates appropriate non-verbal behaviour (e.g. eye contact, posture and position, movement, facial expression, use of voice).

25 Use of notes: if reads, writes notes or uses computer, does so in a manner that does not interfere with dialogue or rapport.

26 Acceptance: acknowledges patient's views and feelings; accepts legitimacy; is not judgemental.

27 Empathy and support: expresses concern, understanding, willingness to help; acknowledges coping efforts and appropriate self-care.

28 Sensitivity: deals sensitively with embarrassing and disturbing topics and physical pain, including when associated with physical examination.

Involving the patient

29 Sharing of thoughts: shares thinking with patient as appropriate to encourage patient's involvement, enhance understanding (e.g. 'What I'm thinking now is that . . .').

30 Provides rationale: explains rationale for questions or parts of physical examination that could appear to be non-sequiturs.

31 Examination: during physical examination, explains processes, asks permission.

Explanation and planning

Providing the correct amount and type of information

Aims: to give comprehensive and appropriate information
    to assess each individual patient's information needs
    to neither restrict nor overload

32 Chunks and checks: gives information in assimilable chunks; checks for understanding, uses patient's response as a guide to how to proceed.

33 Assesses patient's starting point: asks for patient's prior knowledge early on when giving information; discovers extent of patient's wish for information.

34 Asks patient what other information would be helpful (e.g. aetiology, prognosis).

35 Gives explanations at appropriate times: avoids giving advice, information or reassurance prematurely.

Aiding accurate recall and understanding

Aims: to make information easier for the patient to remember and understand

36 Organizes explanation: divides into discrete sections; develops a logical sequence.

37 Uses explicit categorization or signposting (e.g. 'There are three important things that I would like to discuss. First . . .'; 'Now, shall we move on to . . .').

38 Uses repetition and summarizing to reinforce information.

39 Language: uses concise, easily understood statements; avoids or explains jargon

40 Uses visual methods of conveying information: diagrams, models, written information and instructions.

41 Checks patient's understanding of information given (or plans made), e.g. by asking patient to restate in own words; clarifies as necessary.

Achieving a shared understanding: incorporating the patient's perspective

Aims: to provide explanations and plans that relate to the patient's perspective of the problem

to discover the patient's thoughts and feelings about the information given

to encourage an interaction rather than one-way transmission

42 Relates explanations to patient's illness framework: to previously elicited ideas, concerns and expectations.

43 Provides opportunities and encourages patient to contribute: to ask questions, seek clarification or express doubts; responds appropriately.

44 Picks up verbal and non-verbal cues, e.g. patient's need to contribute information or ask questions; information overload; distress.

45 Elicits patient's beliefs, reactions and feelings concerning information given, terms used; acknowledges and addresses where necessary.

Planning: shared decision making

Aims: to allow patient to understand the decision-making process

to involve patient in decision-making to the desired level

to increase the patient's commitment to plans made

46 Shares own thoughts: ideas, thought processes and dilemmas as appropriate.

47 Involves patient by making suggestions rather than imposing directives.

48 Encourages patient to contribute their thoughts: ideas, suggestions and preferences

49 Negotiates a mutually acceptable plan.

50 Offers choices: encourages patient to make choices and decisions to the level they wish.

51 Checks with patient: if plan accepted; if concerns have been addressed.

Closing the session

52 End summary: summarizes session briefly and clarifies plan of care.

53 Contracting: contracts with patient re next steps for patient and physician.

54 Safety net: explains possible unexpected outcomes; what to do if plan is not working; when and how to seek help.

55 Final check: checks that patient agrees and is comfortable with plan and asks if there are any corrections, questions or other items to discuss.

(Source: Silverman, Kurtz and Draper 2004; Kurtz, Silverman and Draper 2004)

Types of doctor–patient relationship

Different models of doctor–patient interactions have been recognized which operate in characteristic ways (Table 6.2). They can be categorized according to the degree of control each party exercises in the encounter:

Paternalistic/consensus

Patient control	Low	High
Doctor control	Low	High

(Patient control: Low underlined; Doctor control: Low underlined)

Paternalistic means 'father-like' although this form of doctor–patient interaction is not unique to male doctors. It is also called the 'consensus' model because it assumes consensus in how the roles should be performed. The power imbalance allows for considerable doctor-centred behaviour – the physician directs and is primarily responsible for decision-making. Poor role-playing (e.g. where there is a rejection of the power dynamics on the part of the patient or their carers) may lead to conflict.

Mutualistic/negotiation

Patient control	Low	High
Doctor Control	Low	High

(Patient control: High underlined; Doctor Control: High underlined)

The mutualistic relationship involves mutual respect in which the patient plays a more active role. The doctor acknowledges the patient's beliefs and knowledge as important, and the outcome of the consultation is the result of a negotiated process of decision-making rather than decisions that are made and imposed by the doctor. The consultation is consequently more participatory and patient-centred.

Consumerist relationship

Patient control	Low	High
Doctor control	Low	High

(Patient control: High underlined; Doctor control: Low underlined)

The consumerist model of doctor–patient interaction is becoming increasingly common in twenty-first-century medicine in the UK. It is based on greater levels of patient choice in whom and when they consult, what to consult about, and the treatments received. With increased access to the internet and other sources of information, patients are becoming more active and demanding of certain treatments (with the doctor's role becoming one of advising and referring on the basis of best available evidence). New types of service delivery, such as drop-in centres, add to the sense of health and health care as commodities that can be 'purchased' much like any other retail item.

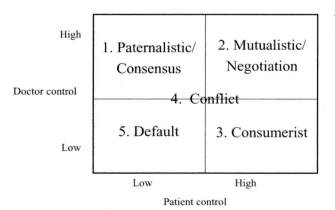

Table 6.2 Types of doctor–patient relationship.

Conflict relationship

Patient control	?	?
Doctor control	?	?

The conflict model is founded on the assumption that doctors and patients inhabit different social worlds. The power imbalance between doctors and patients is contested and leads to conflict. Such conflict may be potential ('latent') or real ('observed'). Conflict that is 'latent' may be revealed subsequently through patient complaints. Routine interactions tend to have elements of both consensus and conflict.

Default relationship

Patient control	Low	High
Doctor control	Low	High

This is an unusual relationship, where neither the doctor nor the patient takes much control. Perhaps the doctor is trying to empower the patient through a patient-centred approach, but the patient doesn't want to take control, so there is lack of engagement (and perhaps conflict) on both sides.

Mutualistic and paternalistic consulting styles compared

There has been much interest in comparing paternalistic and mutualistic relationships in recent years and how doctors may be encouraged to develop a more mutualistic style where appropriate. There is increasing recognition of a spectrum of styles between paternalism and mutualism based on the degree of patient empowerment that is allowed.

Mutualistic = Patient-centred	Paternalistic = Doctor-centred
Marked by high use of:	Marked by high use of:
Open questions (which elicit more than 'yes/no' answers)	Closed questions (which elicit only a yes/no response)
Listening	Questions leading direct to diagnosis
Reflecting	Information gathering
Probing	Analysing
Silence	Disease model – ignoring patient's unique experience
Clarifying	
Facilitating	
Interpreting	
Illness model – incorporating patient's unique experience	

The spectrum from paternalistic to mutualistic consultation styles

Paternalistic	'Doctor knows best', 'directed style'; patient consents to treatment advocated by doctor
Professional as agent	Doctor incorporates patient preferences into decision but makes final decision
Shared model	Process of decision-making and outcome (the decision) both shared
Informed consent model	Doctor provides technical information; patient alone makes the decision

This list shows that consultation styles can vary in the degree of mutualism they demonstrate. The degree of control the patient has in the encounter, as well as the context in which the consultation takes place, determine the style. Sometimes styles can shift even within a consultation. For example, if a patient is unconscious, the paternalistic style will be appropriate. If a doctor is dealing with an elderly patient with chronic rheumatoid arthritis who wants the doctor to decide what to do, then the consultation might start in a paternalistic way but shift to a more shared model over time. Some would argue that in some cases the doctor is defaulting on his or her obligations by making the patient solely responsible for decision-making (as in the informed consent model). However, for some patients suffering from long-term chronic health conditions who have greater knowledge of the condition and/or ways of living with it than the doctor, it may be that this model is the most appropriate.

Doctor–patient relationships in practice

What do patients get, what do they want and who decides?

Studies have shown that patients are more likely to experience a mutualistic consultation if they are younger, have more experience of their condition, are of higher social class and have higher education levels. They are more likely to have a paternalistic consultation if they are older, have less experience of their condition, are from a lower social class and have lower education levels.

Case study: What do patients want?

Patients attending a GP clinic in Scotland were shown ten scripted video vignettes of the decision-making part of a GP consultation, where either a shared decision-making style or a directed style was used. 410 out of 631 (65%) of patients approached agreed to take part in the study. Each of the following five scenarios was scripted in the two different styles:

- Bleeding mole
- Injured leg
- Rheumatoid arthritis
- Depression
- Smoking advice

After watching the pair of vignettes for the particular scenario, patients were asked which they preferred. The researcher found patients varied in their expressed preferences. While there were large minorities in each group holding an opposite viewpoint, the preference for decision-making was associated with:

- The nature of the presenting complaint – patients watching videos of physical problems preferred the directed approach, compared to patients watching a video of a patient with depression.
- The viewer's age – patients aged 60 or more tended to prefer the directed approach.
- The viewer's social class – more patients from social classes 1 and II preferred a shared approach than did those in social classes III–V.
- Smokers preferred a shared approach – perhaps because of prior experiences with overbearing doctors trying to encourage them to stop smoking in a directed way.

There was no significant association found with sex of the patient, frequency of attendance or stated chronic ill health in terms of what kind of style they preferred.

The study concluded that while listening and being open to patients' ideas during the history-taking part of a consultation is vital, patients vary in their desire for involvement in decision-making. It is important that doctors find out how much involvement in decision-making an individual patient actually wants.

Case study: Who decides what patients get?

A Norwegian study published in 1998 compared GPs' consultation styles in dealing with asthma patients. Four styles were identified:

Authoritarian	Teaching	Empowering	Passive
'I will manage it' – adult–child	'I will teach you to manage it' – adult–adolescent	'We will manage it together' – adult–adult	'I do not know how, or even whether, to manage it' – recently qualified and uncertain GPs (= child/adolescent–adult?)

The use of familial relationships as prototypes of doctor–patient relationships (e.g. doctor = adult, patient = child in the 'authoritarian' style) is another useful way of distinguishing different kinds of doctor–patient relationship, although it breaks down somewhat in the 'passive' example above (which was rarely found).

A key finding was that the GP, rather than nature or severity of the illness, determined the management style. Authoritarian doctors tended to have a disease model of asthma and were least likely to take patient or parent knowledge seriously or to treat it with respect. Yet with chronic conditions such as asthma, much of the management of the illness takes place outside the consulting room, and the more authoritarian the medical management, the greater the likelihood of non-compliance/adherence with prescribed treatments.

The benefits of patient-centred medicine

Case study: Seeking fewer repeat consultations by taking patient's fears into account – the case of dyspepsia

Dyspepsia is a major health problem in Britain today; 50% of all adults suffer from recurrent indigestion/heartburn, with 30% of these (i.e. 15% of the adult population) experiencing symptoms every day. Yet studies indicate that dyspepsia, like rectal bleeding, is something of an 'illness iceberg' in medical terms, with less than a third of sufferers likely to have visited their GP during the preceding year regarding their condition. It is estimated that 3–4% of all patients on a GP's list will consult for dyspepsia during any one year. This is a small proportion of those suffering from it, but still represents about 300 consultations per GP a year. Sales of OTC antacids represent one of the largest single sectors of pharmacies' turnover (Chapter 3).

Studies have been conducted into the reasons for consultation with dyspepsia. Contrary to what might be expected, severity and duration of symptoms have relatively little to do with the decision to consult. Rather, it is the beliefs and concerns of the patient that dyspepsia may indicate a serious or potentially life-threatening condition (heart disease, cancer or duodenal ulcer). If the underlying concern is not dealt with and the dyspepsia continues, patients are likely to return to the GP regularly. If GPs arrange the necessary tests in order to check for the underlying illness fear that has triggered a decision to consult, repeat consultations are rarer and patients are generally more satisfied with their treatment.

Figure 6.2 represents the guidelines produced to help doctors manage patients presenting with dyspepsia at general practices in the Middlesbrough area, in 1997. These guidelines were unusual in that they were not focused on identifying the cause of the problem, but on what the patient's concerns were in presenting with the problem. The rationale behind them was that by taking this approach and referring for tests appropriate to the patient's fears, patients would be satisfied and the rate of repeat consultations would decline.

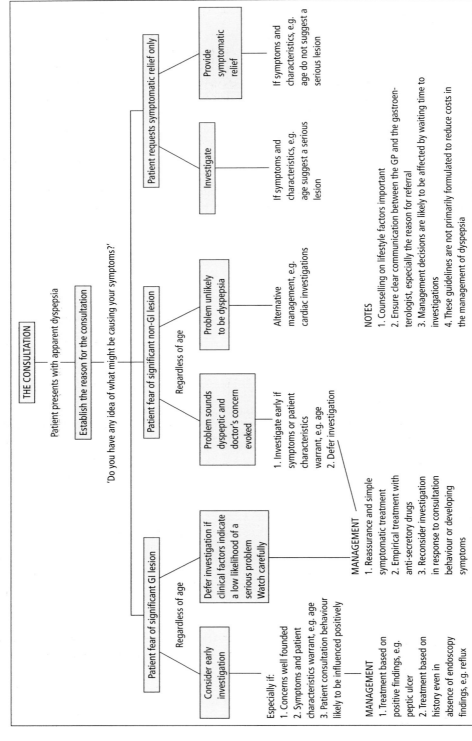

Figure 6.2 Guidelines for the management of patients with dyspepsia (Source: *British Journal of General Practice*, May 1997).

How much is disclosed?

A study of 1470 patients conducted after their GP consultations found that about 60% of patients reporting symptoms in answer to a brief questionnaire had not actually reported some of these in their consultation. Reasons given included:

- Feeling it was not appropriate to ask (36%).
- Feeling hurried (27%).
- Being frightened that the doctor would think less well of them (14%).
- Fear of a bad reaction from the doctor (14%).

The study suggests that a mutualist, patient-centred approach is the way to overcome these barriers.

Does time make a difference?

Patients often complain about lack of time spent with their GP, although average consultation times have almost doubled since 1950. It is not necessarily the case that 'long is good, short is bad'. One study found that average consultations in a general practice lasted eight minutes. When these were increased by one minute for patients presenting with psychosocial problems, this was enough to significantly improve the quality of care. This suggests that, in many cases, while the length of consultation is important, how the time in the consultation is spent is more significant in its impact on the quality of care.

Case study: Whose time? Time pressure in GP consultations

In a study of GP consultations in Buckinghamshire, all patients complained of insufficient time. Although most said they were not rushed and could have asked more questions, most felt guilty about either wasting the doctor's time or taking more than their fair share of time. Thus shortage of time was the major reason given for not asking questions. Typical responses included:

'. . . you're thinking of the person behind you, so you don't want to keep him waiting too long and I wasn't sick, so I'm forgetting the things I want to ask him.'

'You always feel you want to cut corners if you can and get it over as quick as possible so he's not too late finishing because he works so many hours.'

'The only reason I feel guilty is for taking up other people's time . . . I feel personally that, you know, let's hurry up because he's got other people waiting especially sometimes when you go in there and there's four or five people behind you . . .'

What this case study indicates is that perceived time pressure is probably greater for patients than doctors. The power dynamic in the doctor–patient relationship means that even when the patient may overcome the feelings expressed in the above quotes and take time to ask more questions, the doctor has the bulk of the techniques available for ending the consultation at his or her disposal, such as standing up and moving from the chair.

'Ticket of entry' consultations

Some patients present with a condition that is a 'ticket of entry' to a consultation rather than the main problem they want to talk about. Often the 'real' reason for the consultation is revealed in the last few seconds or at the door handle. Whether or not patients disclose their 'real' problems depends on:

- How they perceive the general atmosphere of the consultation.
- Opportunities for sensitive discussion.

Again, a patient-centred, mutualistic consultation which makes patients feel at ease and opens up every opportunity for difficult issues to be discussed is required.

How much clarification is sought?

There are class differences in the extent to which patients seek clarification about their condition. In one study, 27% of working-class patients and 45% of middle-class patients sought clarification. Such questions led to fuller explanations being given by doctors and only slightly longer consultations – in short, a better quality of service.

Concordance: the key to compliance/ adherence outside the clinic

'Compliance' is the old-fashioned word for patients following doctors' instructions and implies a paternalistic approach to patient care. For this reason, 'adherence' is preferable, since it implies a more equal relationship of mutualism. Half of patients with chronic health conditions are estimated not to adhere to their treatment plan, and this can have serious long-term consequences for their health.

Reasons for non-adherence include:
- Forgetting.
- Disagreement with the diagnosis or treatment proposed.
- Side-effects or fear of side-effects.
- Conflict with other aspects of lifestyle.
- Not understanding doctor's advice.
- Distrust/dislike of the doctor and/or dissatisfaction with the consultation.

Communication in a patient-centred way is the key to ensuring maximum adherence to treatment. This means using the consultation as an opportunity to elicit the patient's ideas, concerns and expectations (ICE) about their condition – in other words, their EM – in order to take a shared approach to decision-making. This is known as concordance. Concordance is a quality of the consultation rather than of the patient, while 'non-compliance' and 'non-adherence' can both be used judgementally about patient behaviour. It is possible to have a 'non-concordant' consultation, but not a 'non-concordant' patient.

> **The benefits of patient-centred medicine: a summary**
>
> - More is disclosed.
> - Better handling of 'ticket of entry' consultations.
> - Greater likelihood of clarification being sought.
> - Increased satisfaction.
> - Better concordance, and hence compliance/adherence to treatment outside the clinic.
> - Improved physiological measures.
> - Improved outcomes (e.g. less distress about illness; fewer reported symptoms).
> - Fewer repeat consultations.
> - Reduced costs.

> **Points of view: Choosing the right consulting style for the situation**
>
> Decide which consulting style might be the most appropriate in dealing with each of these clinical situations:
>   Acute infection
>   Chronic illness
>   Coma
>   Delirium
>   Psychotherapy
> What other context-specific situations are likely to influence the nature of the doctor–patient encounter?

New technologies and the doctor–patient encounter

The use of computers and the internet offers new opportunities and challenges for how doctor–patient relationships are managed in the future. Computerized records and information systems threaten to attenuate that 'face-to-face' interactions between doctor and patient which are the strength of the clinical encounter through the doctor having to spend increasing amounts of time looking at a computer monitor during the consultation. The free availability of information about medical conditions on the internet means patients can now arrive at a consultation with sheaves of paper to challenge the doctor's authoritative knowledge. On the other hand, email, text messaging and multi-agent system computing are now widely used in business, leisure and education, and there is no reason in principle why they cannot be extended into the health care domain.

Ways in which internet technologies could improve patient care

Email – clinical advice; ascertaining whether a full consultation might be necessary.
Text messaging – assisting patients with lifestyle choice (e.g. stopping smoking) and medication adherence reminders.
Multi-agent system computing – matching available donor organs to recipient needs for transplant surgery; planning bed usage; booking appointments; ordering prescriptions; obtaining test results; processing simple clinical enquiries.

The main barriers to uptake of these technologies appear to be attitudinal rather than practical, based on concerns about privacy, security and the loss of face-to-face contact. There are justifiable concerns, for example, about safety and confidentiality which have to be addressed before any system can be set up and widely used. There are also concerns that increasing use of internet technology might lead to greater health inequalities because of its limited availability and access among the neediest groups.

Patient and professional experiences of computerised health care

A general practice in Dundee, with a socio-economically mixed patient population of 7000, started using email in 2001 as part of its clinical service, and text messaging in 2004. Over 500 households registered for the services.

A research study was conducted to evaluate how patients and practitioners used and rated the services. Key points to emerge were:

- Email requests for repeat prescriptions were the most frequent use of the facility.
- Text messaging had been slower to take off, largely because of patients' inability to imagine the practical use they might make of it and a perception that this was something better suited to the 'young ones'.
- Patients (including older patients) were generally favourably disposed towards using the services as long as the option for telephone and face-to-face consultation was maintained. As one respondent put it: '*I know that if I ever needed to actually speak to him in person he would always be there*'.
- They also favoured using the service with doctors they had previously met and knew they could trust. One respondent commented: '*I thought, I trust him, so I'll give it a go . . . Maybe if it had been a doctor that I didn't see or I hadn't built up any rapport with then probably I wouldn't have used it*'.
- Respondents generally felt that system security risks were no greater than those for internet shopping or banking, and that the risks were more than outweighed by the benefits of out of hours access and the like.
- Patients and practitioners both appreciated the way in which the technology would have the knock-on benefit of not taking up valuable consultation time with queries that could be answered asynchronously by email. As one respondent commented: '*Last Christmas I got a footbath from my husband but when I read it, it said if you're diabetic consult your doctor. And I thought, I'm going to have to make an appointment to see the doctor for a stupid thing like that. And then I thought, now, I can email. So I did that . . .*'.

Summary

• The consultation is a very structured encounter with many rules and expectations.
• The obligations incumbent on any doctor practising in the UK are enshrined in the GMC's 'Good Medical Practice'.
• Doctors, patients and carers bring different explanatory models to the clinical encounter, and a goal of an effective consultation is to have these converge.
• The Calgary-Cambridge framework for communication is a comprehensive map of communication processes in the consultation. It is important to remember that for effective communication, skills are as dependent on humane practice as on technique.
• Different types of doctor–patient relationship can be identified, on a spectrum from paternalistic to mutualistic.
• The style of consultation chosen is largely determined by the doctor.
• Adoption of a mutualistic, patient-centred approach brings many benefits to both patients and practitioners, and opportunities to make consultations patient-centred should be taken up whenever possible.
• New internet technologies promise to transform elements of the doctor–patient relationship, but trust and face-to-face contact are likely to remain core ingredients.

Further reading

Barry, C. A., Stevenson, F. A., Britten, N., Barber, N. and Bradley, C. P. (2001) Giving voice to the lifeworld. More humane, more effective medical care? A qualitative study of doctor–patient communication in general practice. *Social Science and Medicine*, **53**: 487–505.

Boulton, M., Tuckett, D., Olson, C. and Williams, A. (1986) Social class and the general practice consultation. *Sociology of Health and Illness*, **8(4)**: 325–50.

Brewin, T. B. (1985) Truth, trust and paternalism. *Lancet*, **2(8453)**: 490–2.

Reproduced in B. Davey, Gray, A. and Seale, C. (eds) (1994) *Health and Disease: a Reader* (2nd edn.). Buckingham: Open University Press, pp 327–31.

Carr, J. and Sheikh, A. (2004) E-mail consultations in health care: 1 – scope and effectiveness; 2 – acceptability and safe application. *British Medical Journal*, **329**: 435–8, 439–42.

Cromarty, I. (1996) What do patients think about during their consultations? A qualitative study. *British Journal of General Practice*, **46**: 525–8.

General Medical Council (2006) Good Medical Practice. London: General Medical Council.

Graham, H. and Oakley, A. (1981) Competing ideologies of reproduction: medical and maternal perspectives on pregnancy. In H. Roberts (ed.) *Women, Health and Reproduction*. London: Routledge & Kegan Paul. Reproduced in C. Currer and M. Stacey (eds) (1986) *Concepts of Health, Illness and Disease: a Comparative Perspective*. Oxford: Berg, pp. 99–115.

Henwood, F., Wyatt, S., Hart, A. and Smith, J. (2003) 'Ignorance is bliss sometimes': constraints in the emergence of the 'informed patient' in the changing landscapes of health information. *Sociology of Health and Illness*, **25**: 589–607.

Hungin, A. P. S., Rubin, G. P., Russell, A. and Convery, B. (1997) Guidelines for dyspepsia management in general practice using focus groups. *British Journal of General Practice*, **47(418)**: 275–9.

Kurtz, S. M., Silverman, J. D. and Draper, J. (2004) *Teaching and Learning Communication Skills in Medicine* (2nd rev. edn.). Oxford: Radcliffe Medical Press.

Lagerlov, P., Leseth, A. and Matheson, I. (1998) The doctor–patient relationship and the management of asthma. *Social Science and Medicine*, **47(1):** 85–91.

McKinstry, B. (2000) Do patients wish to be involved in decision making in the consultation? A cross-sectional survey with video vignettes. *British Medical Journal*, **321**: 867–71.

Mullen, P. D. (1997) Compliance becomes concordance. *British Medical Journal*, **314**: 691–2.

Neighbour, R. (2004) *The Inner Consultation: How to Develop an Effective and Intuitive Consulting Style* (2nd rev. edn.). Oxford: Radcliffe Publishing.

Neville, R. G., Greene, A. and Lewis, S. (2006) Patient and health care professional views and experiences of computer agent-supported health care. *Informatics in Primary Care*, **14**: 11–15.

Pendleteon, D. and Bochner, S. (1980) The communication of medical information in GP consultations as a function of social class. *Social Science and Medicine*, **14A**: 669–73.

Pendleton, D., Schofield, T., Tate, P. and Havelock, P. (2003) *The New Consultation: Developing Doctor–Patient Communication* (2nd rev. edn.). Oxford: Oxford University Press.

Potter, S. J. and McKinlay, J. B. (2005) From a relationship to encounter: an examination of longitudinal and lateral dimensions in the doctor–patient relationship. *Social Science and Medicine*, **61(2)**: 465–79.

Seale, C. (1994) Doctor–patient interaction. In C. Seale and S. Pattison (eds) *Medical Knowledge: Doubt and Certainty*. Buckingham: Open University Press.

Shaw, J. and Baker, M. (2004) Expert patient: dream or nightmare? *British Medical Journal*, **328**: 723–4.

Silverman, J. D., Kurtz, S. M. and Draper, J. (2004) *Skills for Communicating with Patients* (2nd rev. edn.). Oxford: Radcliffe Medical Press.

Tuckett, D., Boulton, M., Oban, C. and Williams, A. (1985) *Meetings between Experts: an Approach to Sharing Ideas in Medical Consultations*. London: Tavistock.

Young, B., Dixon-Woods, M., Findlay, M. and Heney, D. (2002) Parenting in a crisis: conceptualising mothers of children with cancer. *Social Science and Medicine,* **55**: 1835–47.

Zola, I. (1973) Pathways to the doctor from person to patient. *Social Science and Medicine*, **7**: 677–89.

Chapter 7

Health inequalities

Introduction

Health and ill health are not randomly distributed across the UK. Health differences exist between places and among different people living in the same place. They are also to be found in more extreme form among countries. Some people refer to these differences as 'health variations', which could be simply the result of genetic differences, geography or chance. Whatever efforts are made, factors such as these mean that full equality in health is not achievable. However, evidence suggests that many health differences are due to factors that are largely socially determined and hence avoidable. These inequalities are reflected in different life expectancy and morbidity between groups. Death as a biological inevitable is very democratic; its deferral, and the quality of life experienced leading up to it, are not. The reasons for these differences are primarily social and economic, not biological. They are of serious concern to society in terms of the wasted potential, economic burden and psychological distress caused by long-standing illness and premature mortality.

The most common way in which health inequalities are measured in the UK is by comparing mortality and morbidity levels by social class, and this is the focus of this chapter. Other variables, such as gender and ethnicity, are discussed in Chapter 8.

This chapter covers the following topics

Ways of measuring social class
Patterns of class-based inequalities in health and health care in the UK
Explanations of class/health differences
Health inequalities at the global level
The medical relevance of health inequalities

Ways of measuring social class

Three measures of social class

1 Registrar-General's classification.
2 The National Statistics Socio-Economic Classification (NS-SEC).
3 Indices of Deprivation.

The Registrar-General's classification

The most common classification of social classes until recently was that used by the Registrar-General. It is based on occupation, ranked according to relative skill, social status and prestige. The five classes distinguished are shown in Table 7.1.

Lecture Notes: *The Social Basis of Medicine*, 1st edition. By Andrew Russell. Published 2009 by Blackwell Publishing. ISBN: 978-1-4051-3912-0

Table 7.1 The Registrar-General's classification of social classes.

Social Class	Title	Examples
I*	Professional	Doctors, lawyers
II*	Intermediate non-manual	Teachers, nurses, most managers and senior administrators
IIIa*	Skilled non-manual	Clerks, shop assistants
IIIb	Skilled manual	Bricklayers, coalminers, bus drivers
IV	Semi-skilled manual	Bus conductors, postal workers
V	Unskilled manual	Porters, cleaners, labourers

*Indicates 'non-manual' class; the rest are 'manual' (Source: National Statistics website http://www.statistics.gov.uk)

Some problems with the Registrar-General's classification of social classes

• Occupation is being used as a proxy for social class.

• Occupation is not always a good reflection of levels of income or poverty. A professional footballer, for example (a skilled non-manual occupation), can earn millions of pounds or very little. Less extreme examples of such variation can be found in many other occupation groups.

• The Registrar-General's classification often leads to inaccurate measurement of social status in certain groups, such as the retired.

• Women who live with a male partner or parent are classified according to the occupation of the partner or parent, not their own occupation.

• The unemployed are classified by their occupation when employed, which may not represent their current status or income.

• Social class is about more than just occupation. Lay people tend to make crude distinctions between the 'middle classes' (non-manual groups) and 'working classes' (manual groups), but also more subtle distinctions based on education, income, location, accent, attitudes, beliefs and behaviour in their assessment of a person's position in society.

• Social class is being used as a proxy for a range of factors which might more directly influence health, such as education, income, housing and behaviour. In other countries these are often used as the primary measure when looking at inequalities in heath.

Despite these provisos, social class determined on the basis of occupation as defined by the Registrar-General remains a powerful predictor of health risks and outcomes.

The National Statistics Socio-Economic Classification (NS-SEC)

The NS-SEC was introduced in 2001 with the intention of establishing a more meaningful, occupation-based classification by focusing on employment relations and conditions rather that skill and prestige. It divides the adult population into eight categories (Table 7.2). Some differences from the Registrar-General's classification include excluding the retired and long-term unemployed from the analysis. The eight classes can be aggregated into three (managerial/professional; intermediate; routine and manual) which roughly correspond with the non-manual/manual distinction of the Registrar-General (Table 7.1).

The findings from studies that have compared morbidity and mortality data according to the Registrar-General's classification with that of the new NS-SEC classification show that, while substantial differences across the social scale remain, the social gradient for adult mortality is not always so clear.

Indices of Deprivation

This classifier is based on measurements of the level of 'deprivation' (or affluence) of the area where people live as a proxy for their social class. The version most commonly used in England is the Indices of Deprivation 2004 (ID 2004). Figures have been generated for 32,482 Super Output Areas (SOAs; areas smaller than Local Authorities) in England. The seven domains on which the index is based, with their relative weightings, are indicated in Table 7.3.

Table 7.2 The eight class grouping of the National Statistics Socio-economic classification (Source: National Statistics website http://www.statistics.gov.uk).

Classification title	Description	Examples of occupations
1 Higher managerial and professional occupations	This includes employers in large organizations, managerial professions and higher professional occupations. Higher managerial professions are those which involve general planning and supervision of operations on behalf of an employer.	Doctors Lawyers Dentists Professors Professional engineers
2 Lower managerial and professional occupations	This includes lower professional and higher technical occupations, lower managerial occupations and higher supervisory occupations.	School teachers Nurses Journalists Actors Police sergeants
3 Intermediate occupations	These are positions in clerical, sales and intermediate technical occupations that do not involve general planning or supervisory powers.	Airline cabin crew Secretaries Photographers Firemen Auxiliary nurses
4 Small employers and own account workers	Small employers are those, other than higher or lower professionals, who employ others and so assume some degree of control over them. These employers carry out all or most of the entrepreneurial and managerial functions of the enterprise. Own account workers are self-employed people engaged in any (non-professional) trade, personal service or semi-routine, routine or other occupation but have no employees other than family workers.	Non-professionals with fewer than 25 employees e.g. self-employed builders, hairdressers of fishemen Shopkeepers – own own shop

Category	Description	Examples
5 Lower supervisory and technical occupations	Lower supervisory occupations have titles such as 'foreman' and 'supervisor' and have formal and immediate supervision over those in classes 6 and 7. Lower technical occupations are technical jobs which have some service elements in their employment contracts (for example, work autonomy).	Train drivers Employed plumbers or electricians Foremen Supervisors
6 Semi-routine occupations	The work involved requires at least some element of employee discretion/ decision making.	Shop assistants Postmen Security guards Call centre workers Care assistants
7 Routine occupations	Positions with a basic labour contract, in which employees are paid for the specific service. Employee discretion/decision making less relevant here.	Bus drivers Waitresses Cleaners Car park attendants Refuse collectors
8 Never worked and long-term unemployed	People in this category have never had an occupation or have been unemployed for an extended period and can therefore not be assigned to an NS-SEC category. 'Long-term' can be defined as any period of time but is generally one or two years. In the Labour Force Survey it is one year or longer.	
Not classified (including full-time students, occupations not stated or inadequately described and not classified for other reasons)	Occupations not stated or inadequately classified are those where there is insufficient information to classify the individual. Not classifiable for other reasons includes, for example, the retired, long-term sick and disabled, people looking after the home and short term unemployed when a previous occupation cannot be found. Full-time students are normally recorded as students even if a previous occupation is given.	

For more information on NS-SEC see *The National Statistics Socio-economic Classification: User Manual.*

Table 7.3 The seven domains of the Indices of Deprivation 2004

Domain	Weighting	Examples of indicators
Income deprivation	22.5%	Adults and children in income support households
Employment deprivation	22.5%	Unemployment benefit claimants
		'New Deal' participants
Health deprivation and disability	13.5%	Measures of emergency admissions to hospital
		Adults under 60 suffering from mood or anxiety disorders
Education, skills and training deprivation	13.5%	Average points score of children at different 'Key Stages'
		Proportion of working-age adults with no or low qualifications
Barriers to housing and services	9.3%	Household overcrowding
		Road distance to GP, supermarket, primary school and Post Office
Crime	9.3%	Rates of burglary, theft, criminal damage and violence
Living environment and deprivation	9.3%	Houses without central heating
		Air quality

The main advantage of using the Indices of Deprivation is that all that is needed to allocate class is a postcode. Since these (unlike occupation) are found on many routine health datasets, it makes the Indices easier to use. The main disadvantage is that no area, however small, is homogeneous (e.g. there may be multiple-occupation houses in an affluent area, or houses in good condition on a council estate, for example), so some individuals will be misclassified. This is known as the 'ecological fallacy' and means that index of deprivation scores based on location are an even more remote proxy for 'social class' than measures based on occupation.

Patterns of class-based inequalities in health and health care in the UK

Types of health inequality

- Inequalities in mortality
- Inequalities in morbidity
- Inequalities in health care: the 'inverse care law'

Inequalities in mortality

Figure 7.1 shows that, despite the improvements in health in the UK as a whole, mortality rates among men of different social classes are widening rather than narrowing. Similarly the infant mortality rate among the manual class groups, was 13% higher than for the total population in 1997–99, but in 2001–3, it had increased to 19%. However, differences in general heart disease and cancer mortality rates seem to be narrowing.

Mortality in classes I and V, the 'twice as likely' comparisons

- In Britain in 2000, infant mortality in social class V was twice that of social class I.
- Child mortality for 15 year olds in social class V was twice that of those in social class I.
- British men in social class V are more than twice as likely to die before retirement age than those in social class I.

Stop Press! The major air crash comparison

The 'excess deaths' among people aged 16–74 in the manual compared to the non-manual classes in the UK is the same as would result from a jumbo jet crashing every day. Yet this excess is rarely commented on in the media. Is this because it is regarded as inevitable or unavoidable?

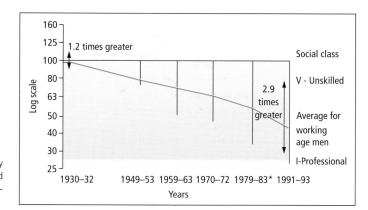

Figure 7.1 The widening mortality gap between classes: 1930–32 and 1991–93 compared (Source: Department of Health 2003).

Are some kinds of death more common among non-manual than manual groups?

A popular stereotype is of a hard-nosed, driven and wealthy businessman dropping dead prematurely with a heart attack. Psychologists have identified a Type A behaviour pattern and have hypothesized that it is linked to susceptibility to particular illnesses.

The three components identified in the Type A behaviour pattern are:

1 Competitive achievement orientation

2 Time urgency

3 Easy arousal to anger/hostility

Hypothesized associations of Type A behaviour with asthma and indigestion have not been proved, but various studies have indicated an association between Type A behaviour and coronary heart disease (CHD). It seems that easy arousal to anger and hostility are the key variables linked to increased propensity to CHD, due to the stress-related hormone levels of people who are frequently hostile (see Chapter 8). However, the relationship between Type A behaviour and social class is unclear.

It could be that the lay perception of CHD as a killer disease of the non-manual classes has some basis in history, since the mortality rate was highest in social class I and lowest in social class V for the first half of the twentieth century, only reversing in the final quarter century. However if one looks at 'causes of death' from death certificates it turns out that in 80% of cases a particular cause is found more commonly in the manual than the non-manual classes. Of the 14 major categories used by the International Classification of Diseases, only malignant melanoma for men and four diseases (including breast cancer) for women reverse this pattern.

Inequalities in morbidity

Morbidity rates are similarly unequally distributed, although are more difficult to measure accurately. Consultation rates are higher for manual than non-manual workers, but this could also be due to differences in health-seeking behaviour (see Chapter 3). Self-reported illness rates are also higher among manual compared to non-manual groups, particularly rates of chronic illness and disability. These differences widen among older age groups, which is significant since the social class gradient in mortality rates tends to narrow with age.

Inequalities in health care: the 'inverse care law'

In 1971, Julian Tudor Hart, a GP practising in South Wales, published his 'inverse care law' which states that 'the availability of good medical care tends to vary inversely with the need of the population served'. While cleverly phrased, and still widely quoted, this is an observation rather than a law. 'Class-marked' differences in services have been observed in the following areas:

- Availability or accessibility of services.
- Standards of premises, equipment and training.
- Quality of service (e.g. length of consultation, number of problems discussed, information given; see Chapter 6).
- Access to information.
- Use of preventive services (e.g. presentation for antenatal supervision and postnatal examination; immunizations, uptake of vitamin supplements; screening services).

There have been many studies to substantiate Tudor Hart's observation over the last quarter of a century, but there are also studies showing services well targeted to need, such as smoking cessation in the North East of England. There is a danger that by treating Tudor Hart's observation as a 'law' people will assume it always applies and is an inevitable, foregone conclusion.

Case study: The resource allocation formula in the NHS

The NHS currently has a resource allocation formula which links resources to identified need. It contains a health inequalities adjustment in an attempt to target more resources to areas of highest health inequality. (There are numerous arguments as to how much extra money is needed for a given inequality in health or need.) It is administered through the Primary Care Trusts and covers hospital and community health services and prescribing. However, it is one thing to have resources allocated and another to actually be able to use these resources in areas of greatest need. For example, even when a practice is open, it can be difficult to recruit GPs to work in areas of high socioeconomic deprivation. However, as a result of this formula there has been a reduction in regional inequalities in the geographical distribution of doctors. It takes time for increased expenditure to make a difference to health outcomes, but some of the most recent studies are starting to find that, as a result of appropriately targeted services, health outcomes in areas demonstrating the highest inequalities are improving.

Explanations of class/health differences

Four types of explanation for class and health differences in the UK

1 Artefact
2 Social selection/mobility
3 Cultural/behavioural
4 Materialist

Artefact

These are explanations suggesting that the differences can be put down to technical issues in measurement (i.e. how the statistics are collected and used). Such differences can be of two sorts:

- Numerator–denominator bias.
- Changes in group size.

Numerator–denominator bias

One example is when death certificate registration is used to show the number of deaths in each social class while Census information is used to find the number of individuals in each class. People's occupations might be described differently in the two forms of data collection. Census data are self-provided, and it may be that some people 'inflate' their occupational status. If this makes it appear that there are fewer people in the lower social classes, this will make it seem that the mortality rate in the lower classes is higher.

Changes in group size

The reduction in the number of manual jobs due to the increasing use of technology has led to fewer people being classified in social classes IV and V. Those remaining in social class V may be those who are at greater risk of dying. Thus comparisons over time might make it appear that health inequalities remain the same or are increasing when in fact they are declining.

While one must always be cautious of the potential for statistics to mislead, neither of these two explanations has stood up to close scrutiny. Longitudinal studies of smaller sample groups have been conducted that have ensured individuals are classified at death as in the same social class as they were in an earlier Census. These have found differences in mortality remain broadly similar to those that use both Census and death certificate data, with only a small degree of artefactual bias detectable. Others have suggested that, far from over-emphasizing health inequalities, artefactual explanations may actually underestimate them. For example, measures other than standardized mortality ratios (e.g. those that take the number of life years lost) indicate greater differences between the social classes than do measures where age is controlled for.

Social selection/mobility

The social selection/mobility explanation asks which comes first – class or ill health. Rather than social class determining health, could health not be a determinant of an individual's social class, so that those who are healthy move up through the social classes, while those who are unhealthy move down?

There is evidence that this is true for some chronic conditions (e.g. epilepsy, schizophrenia and bronchitis). However, social selection/mobility cannot explain the class gradient in infant mortality, since infants have not had the opportunity to move up or down the class ladder. Sociological studies indicate that social mobility has more to do with education, family attitudes and changes in

the social structure (e.g. the rise in non-manual, 'white-collar' jobs) than with health.

Cultural/behavioural

These are the explanations that suggest it is class differences in attitudes, beliefs and behaviour (e.g. about health in general, or smoking) that cause most of the inequalities in health. For example, a middle-class, 'idealist' view of health (see Chapter 2) is likely to prompt earlier consultations and greater use of preventive services than a 'functional' view of health.

Cultural/behavioural explanations tend to be the basis of much health promotion work, based on the assumption that these beliefs and behaviours are to a certain extent the subject of individual education and/or choice, and hence can be changed. The four main health-related behaviours targeted are smoking, alcohol consumption, diet and exercise. However, in adopting this approach there is the danger of stereotyping or stigmatizing people's ways of life and their accompanying beliefs and behaviour – a 'blame the victim' mentality. Much of the apparently 'chosen' behaviour that is the object of health promotion is, on more careful investigation, not freely chosen at all. For example, studies of dietary habits have shown that food preferences are culturally embedded, and food availability (irrespective of preference) is linked to disposable income.

Case study: Smoking – a major behavioural risk factor

There are more male and female smokers in social class V than in social class I, and they are less likely to give up their habit successfully (Figure 7.2). It is estimated that half the difference in survival to 70 years of age between people in social class V and social class I is attributable to smoking.

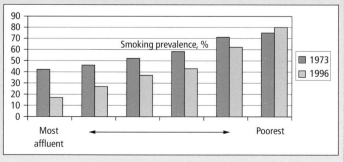

Figure 7.2 Smoking by deprivation, Great Britain, 1973 and 1996 (Source: Derek Wanless, Department of Health Tackling Health Inequalities summit, 17–18 October 2005).

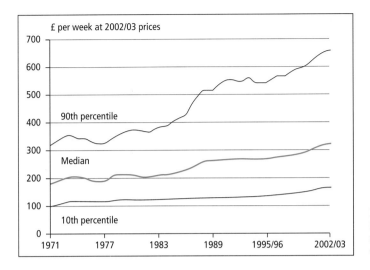

Figure 7.3 Distribution of real household disposable income in the UK (Source: National Statistics website: www.statistics.gov.uk).

Materialist

Materialist explanations focus on the living and working conditions of people in the different social classes, factors over which they have little or no control. Key factors identified include income, housing and the work environment.

Income

Income may be derived from a variety of sources: employment, interest on savings, welfare benefits, pensions (which are frequently linked to pay levels when in work). As well as amount of income, regularity of payment and how it is distributed within the household are important in determining its likely effects on health. The gap in the average weekly income between the highest and lowest percentiles has increased from just over 1:3 in 1971 to nearly 1:4 in 2002–3 (Figure 7.3).

Wealth (i.e. assets as well as income) is currently even more unequally distributed. Half the population of the UK owned just 8 per cent of the wealth in 1976, but this had declined to 5 per cent in 2001.

Debt levels are also high in the UK. About one third of adults have unsecured personal loans, overdrafts and credit card debts greater than they expect to be able to pay off at the end of the month, and 13% of debtors in 2003 owed £10,000 or more. Debt can be a source of considerable psychological strain.

Case study: Welfare rights advice in general practice

In 1999, the Middlesbrough Welfare Rights Unit initiated a project with the local Primary Care Trust to give welfare benefits advice to people who were assessed to be in need of it in all the general practices in the city. The scheme currently employs three welfare rights workers (one full-time and two part-time). They hold six outreach surgeries a week in the six main GP clinics and also staff a telephone advice line. In 2006–7, they helped 348 patients get £829,892 in unclaimed benefits to which they were entitled – an average of £2,378 per client!

Delivering welfare rights advice in health care settings is becoming more common in the UK and, as the above example shows, can have profound financial implications for the individuals concerned. It is difficult, however, to gather information about what the measurable long-term health or social benefits of such interventions might be. Given the importance of the link between income and health, however, it can be assumed that initiatives such as this should play an important part in the health and social care provided by general practices in the future.

Housing

Many aspects of housing can affect health:

Location: including noise levels, air pollution, availability of services such as shops, transport and safe play areas, levels of crime and vandalism.

Design and maintenance of housing: cost of heating, damp, condensation, vermin (e.g. rats, insects), electrical and other fire hazards, availability of safe play space.

Overcrowding/multiple occupation: some families have to share bathrooms, toilets and kitchens; sanitation and fire escapes inadequate for numbers. In 2006, more than 500,000 households were estimated to be living in overcrowded conditions.

All these issues are more common among people in social classes IV and V than social classes I, II and III. Respiratory diseases in children and young people can be particularly affected by housing quality. It was estimated that, in 2006, 728,000 homes in the UK were 'officially unfit for human habitation'.

Work environment

There are a number of ways in which the work environment can impact on health:

Pay: 60% of manual workers were paid an hourly rate of £5 or less in 1989, compared to 20% of non-manual workers; no manual workers were paid more than £11 per hour in 1989, compared to 20% of non-manual workers.

Hours worked: people in manual work tend to work longer hours and do more overtime than non-manual workers.

Shift work: manual workers are more likely to do shift work, often at unsociable hours.

Quality of the work environment: noise, likelihood of accidents, exposure to toxic substances – all are greater among manual compared to non-manual groups.

Autonomy: manual workers, particularly those on production lines, tend to have less control over the tempo and organization of their work. Lack of control is recognized as a source of stress.

Redundancy: more likely among manual workers than non-manual workers.

Financial planning: more difficult for manual workers given the uncertainties in their working lives.

Poverty

Poverty is an extreme and all-embracing form of deprivation where the material, cultural and social resources are so limited that the individuals, families and groups affected find themselves excluded from the minimum acceptable standard of living of the country in which they are located. According to the WHO, poverty is the leading cause of ill health in the world today.

Poverty can be measured in the following ways
- In absolute terms (e.g. when linked to 'basic needs').
- In relative terms (e.g. relative to the rest of society).
- By degree of social exclusion.
- Longitudinally.

All these measures tend to be greater among ethnic minorities, the disabled, the chronically sick, single people and the elderly. The numbers experiencing poverty in their lifetimes is almost always greater than those measured in a snapshot view and can often be a 'hidden factor' in current health problems.

Poverty in the UK is often associated with:
- Homelessness, or the threat of it.
- Unemployment (worklessness).

Homelessness

There are two types of homeless people: the official homeless and those who are unofficial homeless.

Official homeless people are legally recognized as having nowhere to live under the 1985 Housing Act. The responsibility of local authorities is to place them in (often temporary) accommodation. They are mainly couples with children, single parents, pregnant women or those who are vulnerable because of mental illness or disability.

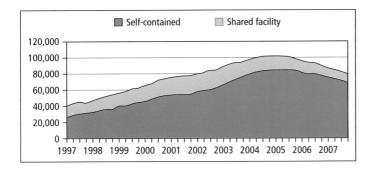

Figure 7.4 Households in England in temporary accommodation at the end of each quarter, by type (Source: Communities and Local Government website: http://www.communities.gov.uk).

Numbers of official homeless fluctuate over time: 73% of households in temporary accommodation in 2006 included dependent children (Figure 7.4).

The *unofficial homeless* are people not officially registered as homeless who sleep on the streets or in night shelters, hostels or other accommodation (e.g. friends' floors, campsites). They are mainly single, unemployed white adult males. They often lack educational qualifications and may have spent time in institutions (children's homes, prisons or general or psychiatric hospitals). How many people fall into the category of 'unofficial homeless' is uncertain and are hotly contested, but may be as high as 380,000 in the UK.

Unemployment

Unemployment and ill health could be an artefact (e.g. if people who are unemployed have more motivation to become defined as 'ill') or the result of social selection (if ill health is the cause rather than the result of unemployment). However, longitudinal studies of people who lost employment for reasons unrelated to ill health have shown convincingly that unemployment is itself a cause of ill health, particularly if the unemployment is prolonged, for the following reasons:

- The significant *material* effects of unemployment (e.g. on diet and housing).
- The contribution of unemployment to higher levels of *stress* and *demoralization.*
- The *isolation* unemployment causes people from the strong and supportive social relationships found in many workplaces

Psychosocial explanations of health inequalities

During the 1990s, research provided additional perspectives on the materialist explanations of health inequalities. This work suggested that it is the psychological influence of social status associated with particular levels of income that is crucial in explaining health inequalities. A greater level of hierarchy and inequality in developed societies threatens social cohesion and produces more social conflict. It has also been shown that there is a relationship not just between income and health, but also between the width of income inequality and mortality rates.

Studies of Whitehall civil servants in the 1980s and 1990s showed a steady gradient in mortality among the different grades of the male civil servant population (Figure 7.5). The age-standardized mortality over a ten-year period of male civil servants aged 40–64 was about 3½ times higher for those in the clerical and manual grades compared to the senior administrative grades.

While incomes differ, none of the individuals concerned could be said to be materially deprived or living in poverty – there are no 'have-nots', except in status. The main differences between them come from the levels of control they exert and autonomy they enjoy in the workplace, the monotony of the tasks they have to perform, the level of support they receive from their peers and their relationship with superiors.

Support and relationship quality are examples of the buffer effect on health inequalities that may be provided by community ties and social cohesion – the value of what has come to be called 'social capital'.

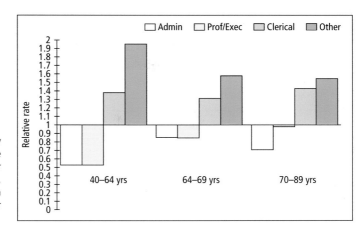

Figure 7.5 All causes of mortality by grade of employment – male Whitehall civil servants followed for 25 years (Source: Derek Wanless, Department of Health Tackling Health Inequalities summit, 17–18 October 2005).

Case study: Baboons and civil servants – can primatology provide a key?

Possible biological pathways to explain the differential mortality between grades of civil servant are hinted at by studies of primate hierarchies. Olive baboons in the Serengeti, for example, form hierarchies much like British civil servants. Physiological measurements of baboons indicate that low-ranking males have much higher levels of glucocorticoids than high-ranking ones. (Glucocorticoids are released during stress as part of the 'fight or flight' hormone response of subordinate males as they are constantly 'faced down' by the more dominant ones.)

This physiological response to stress is turned off more rapidly in dominant males after the stressful event has passed. In other words, subordinate baboons are in a continuous state of low-level readiness or anxiety. The only time that the superior functioning of the endocrine system of the dominant males is impaired is when the dominance hierarchy is disrupted and, with status uncertain, all animals begin to show the continuing anxiety and low-level stress response characteristic of subordinates.

The physiological and mental responses to prolonged stress are known to have deleterious effects on a number of biological systems and to give rise to a number of illnesses. Similar results have been found in blood pressure measurements taken from high- and low-grade civil servants both at work and at home. The blood pressure of all ranks is elevated at work, but when they go home the blood pressure of senior administrators drops much more rapidly. It seems they are better able to turn off the 'stress response' (although some critics have suggested that the home environment of the senior civil servants may also be more conducive to 'destressing'). There is also an inverse relationship between grade of civil servant and levels of fibrinogen circulating in the blood (fibrinogen is a risk factor in cardiovascular disease). It need not be that the 'stress response' of either low-status baboons or civil servants is inappropriate, and could be learned. A low-ranking baboon never knows when a higher-ranking animal is going to drive him away from a meal or a female. This 'learned helplessness', characterized in humans by a sense of melancholy, lethargy and inadequacy, is a common response to an unsatisfactory social environment.

Health inequalities at the global level

Inequalities in health between countries are even starker than they are within countries. For example, it is estimated that the 225 richest people in the world have the same amount of assets as the poorest 2.5 billion have in income. More than half of all household wealth in the world is owned by the richest 2% of the adult population, whereas the 50% of people at the bottom end of the scale, financially speaking, own barely 1% of the global household wealth. 1.3 billion people live on less than US$1 a day; in contrast, it is estimated that every cow in the EU is subsidized to the tune of US$2.5 a day. Health expenditure per capita in the UK is $3000; in Malawi it is $12.

Just as the health of the working classes contrasts with that of the middle and upper classes in the UK, so the health statistics of people in less developed countries (LDCs) compare unfavourably with those in more developed countries (MDCs). There is also much variation within countries. No country has been found where inequalities are absent, although some (e.g. in Scandinavia) have much smaller gaps than others (e.g. in North America). Evidence suggests that, given two countries of equivalent Gross Domestic Product (GDP), the more equal the income distribution in each country, the better their average level of health, particularly in early to middle adulthood.

> *More developed countries* include all countries in Europe, North America, Australia, New Zealand and Japan.
> *Less developed countries* include all countries in Africa, Asia (excluding Japan), Latin America and the Caribbean, and the regions of Melanesia, Micronesia and Polynesia (South Pacific).

Age-specific mortality at the global level

The major difference between the two lines in Figure 7.6 is the much higher rate of infant mortality in Egypt. After that, the lines are much more similar, if consistently somewhat higher in Egypt than in England and Wales.

Infant mortality at the global level

Figure 7.7 shows the stark contrasts in infant mortality rates in different parts of the world, while Figures 7.8 and 7.9 show the improvements made in most countries in the second half of the twentieth century. Poverty is the key to accounting for these differences. Poverty is the result of a variety of factors, usually working together. The WHO identifies the following:

- Lack of income and assets (e.g. food, medicine, education, land and the nurturance of social relationships).
- Isolation (e.g. from water sources, infrastructure such as roads).
- Vulnerability (to outside forces as well as personal circumstances).
- Powerlessness (e.g. to get out of debt; negotiate a decent wage).
- Physical weakness (often caused by poverty, leading to greater poverty).

The 'diseases of poverty' in the LDCs include:

- Infectious diseases (e.g. measles).
- Parasitic diseases (e.g. malaria).
- Respiratory diseases (e.g. tuberculosis).
- Problems at childbirth.

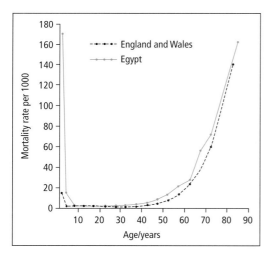

Figure 7.6 Age-specific mortality rates of males in Egypt (1976) and England and Wales (1979) (Source: United Nations Demographic Yearbook 1981).

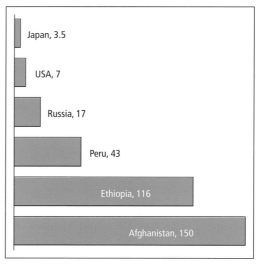

Figure 7.7 Infant mortality rates in selected countries, 2000 (Source: Haub and Cornelius, *2000 World Population Data Sheet*. Washington, DC: Population Reference Bureau).

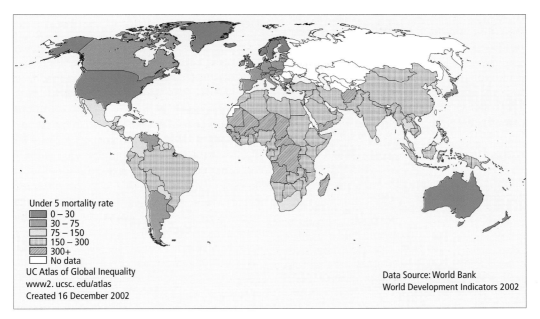

Figure 7.8 1960 mortality rates, under five years old (Source: UC Atlas of Global Inequality: http://ucatlas.ucsc.edu/).

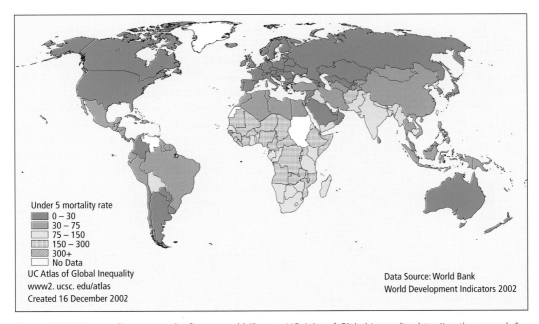

Figure 7.9 2000 mortality rates, under five years old (Source: UC Atlas of Global Inequality: http://ucatlas.ucsc.edu/).

Underlying all these diseases of poverty is a more fundamental 'big killer': malnutrition. The WHO estimates that more than half the deaths represented in Figure 7.10 were associated with malnutrition.

Case study: Global spending on health research

Global spending on health research is skewed towards wealthier nations and their health problems rather than the more pressing problems, in health and survival terms, faced by the poorer countries. Research is also focused on curative medicine rather than prevention. In 1990–2001, the estimated annual expenditure on health research worldwide increased more than three-fold, from £16 billion to £56 billion. This was fairly evenly balanced between the commercial sector (48% – principally the pharmaceutical industry) and the public sector (44 % – including the US National Institutes of Health [NIH], which contributed an average of 20% of the annual total). The remaining 8% came from substantial private, not-for-profit sources, foundations and charities (e.g. the Bill and Melinda Gates Foundation). Research and development is dominated by just a few countries, with the US accounting for nearly half of the total, followed by Japan (13%) and the UK (7%).

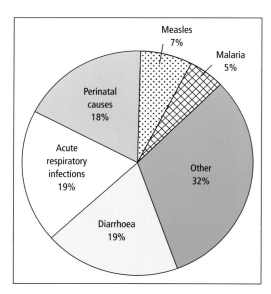

Figure 7.10 Death of children under age of five by main cause, LDCs, 1995 (Source: Haub and Cornelius, *2000 World Population Data Sheet*. Washington, DC: Population Reference Bureau).

The medical relevance of health inequalities

The health inequalities that exist at all levels – local, regional, national and global – are like background music in every doctor's professional career. But, like background music anywhere, with time one can become desensitized and cease to notice it. The Royal College of Physicians has called for doctors to take on a greater role in leadership and community advocacy in society. However, in order to do this doctors need to have a leadership vision and understanding of what they should be advocating, and for whom. Tackling health inequalities through the social and economic determinants of ill health is an obvious remit. One can either do nothing and watch health inequalities grow and be reproduced in future generations, or become involved in attempts to 'level the playing field' of income and resources, which will have a far more profound effect on health than curative medicine alone can ever achieve. Both are essentially political acts.

Good primary care has a key role to play in reducing health inequalities through:
- Providing services that are nearer to people and accessible.
- Focusing on the whole person and their health problems.
- Providing a broad range of services in one setting.
- Coordinating all aspects of care.

In order to be able to provide for the whole person, it is important that the physician has knowledge of the social context, the neighbourhood and community in which the individual lives. Gathering this information at an early stage and continuing to build up knowledge in this way ensures health care can be made appropriate for and targeted at those who need it most.

Summary

- Health is not randomly distributed within and between populations.
- Inequalities in health exist at the local, regional, national and international levels.

- Social class by occupation is a good predictor of health risks and outcomes, and hence health inequalities, for many diseases in the UK.
- Within the UK, the health of the population as a whole has improved, but those in the higher social classes have benefited more from this improvement than those in the manual classes. Inequalities in life expectancy and rates of disease still persist and in some cases are increasing.
- Explanations for health inequalities vary, but materialist explanations appear to be the most powerful.
- At the global level, inequalities in health within and between countries are even starker than health inequalities within the UK.
- Health inequalities provide a challenging agenda for doctors to follow throughout their careers.

Further reading

Adams, J., White, M., Moffatt, S., Howel, D. and Mackintosh, J. (2006) A systematic review of the health, social and financial impacts of welfare rights advice delivered in healthcare settings. *BMC Public Health*, **2006(6)**: 81.

Department of Health (2003) *Tackling Health Inequalities: a Programme for Action*. London: Department of Health.

Dorling, D., Mitchell, R. and Pearce, J. (2007) The global impact of income inequality on health by age: an observational study. *British Medical Journal*, **335**: 873–5.

Leon, D. and Walt, G. (eds) (2001) *Poverty, Inequality and Health: an International Perspective*. Oxford: Oxford University Press.

Marmot, M. (2004) *Status Syndrome: How Your Social Standing Directly Affects Your Health and Life Expectancy*. London: Bloomsbury.

Natarajan, M., Walrond, S. and Chappel, D. (2005) Are NHS stop smoking services reducing health inequalities in the North East of England? *North East Public Health Observatory Occasional Paper No. 20*. Stockton: NEPHO. http://www.nepho.org.uk/index.php?c=1095.

Royal College of Physicians (2005) *Doctors in Society: Medical Professionalism in a Changing World*. London: Royal College of Physicians.

Shaw, M., Davey Smith, G. and Dorling, D. (2005) Health inequalities and New Labour: how the promises compare with real progress. *British Medical Journal*, **330**: 1016–21.

Tudor Hart, J. (1971) The inverse care law. *Lancet*, **1**: 405–12.

Victor, C. (1997) The health of homeless people: a review. *European Journal of Public Health*, **7**: 398–404.

Watt, G. (2002) The inverse care law today. *Lancet,* **360(9328)**: 252–4.

Wilkinson, R. (1996) *Unhealthy Societies: the Afflictions of Inequality*. London: Routledge.

Chapter 8

Sex and gender, race and ethnicity in health and health care

Introduction

Class (Chapter 7) is not the only social category linked to inequalities in health. Inequalities are also manifested in gender, ethnicity, age and disability. In all these, biological and socio-cultural influences work in complex ways to influence health outcomes. This chapter introduces gender and ethnicity as two important determinants of the perceptions and experience of health and health care an individual or a group is likely to have.

This chapter covers the following topics

Sex and gender – what's the difference?
Gender differences in health and illness
Race and ethnicity – what's the difference?
Ethnic differences in health and illness
Cultural competency

Sex and gender – what's the difference?

Sex refers to the anatomical or chromosomal categories of male and female – the biologically given. *Gender* refers to people's socially acquired psychological and cultural characteristics – their culturally ascribed masculinity and femininity.

Lecture Notes: *The Social Basis of Medicine*, 1st edition. By Andrew Russell. Published 2009 by Blackwell Publishing. ISBN: 978-1-4051-3912-0

While almost all people (around 99%) are born biologically male or female, differences between men and women are about more than just differences in biology. Biologically speaking, the differences between men and women are small compared to the similarities in terms of body function and anatomy. There is a tendency to assume that the differences we observe derive from biology. However, even characteristics that we may think of as being linked to hormonal or other physiological influences (e.g. 'sex drive' or 'maternal instinct') are as much a product of social conditioning (socialization) as of biology. The same is true of people's experience of health and illness. Unpicking the relative influence of 'sex' and 'gender' in understanding differences between men and women in terms of health status and uptake of health care is difficult but important, since the assumption that differences are automatically to do with 'biology' often leads to nothing being done about them because they are seen as impossible to change.

Gender differences in health and illness

The basic difference between men and women in their experience of health and illness can be summed up in the grim adage 'women get sick and men die'. At every age in the UK, men have higher mortality rates than women, but women

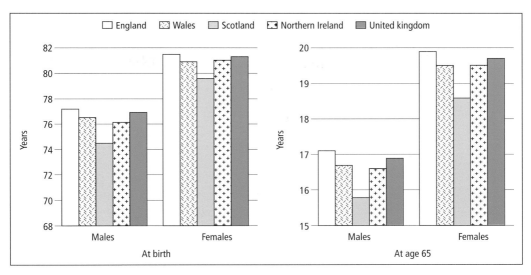

Figure 8.1 Life expectancy in the UK, 2004–6 (Source: National Statistics: www.statistics.gov.uk).

Table 8.1 Self-reported morbidity statistics, UK, 2005 (Source: General Household Survey 2005).

Males, all ages	Females, all ages
Percentage of persons reporting long-standing illness (limiting or non-limiting)	
32	33
Percentage of persons reporting limiting long-standing illness	
18	21
Percentage of persons reporting restricted activity in the 14 days before interview	
11	15
Number of restricted activity days caused by acute sickness in previous year	
24	31

have higher morbidity rates. Figures produced by the National Statistics Office in 2007 show that life expectancy at birth in the UK is 76.9 years for boys and 81.3 years for girls, the highest levels ever recorded (Figure 8.1).

However, while women live longer than men, they suffer from greater morbidity.

Table 8.1 indicates more self-reported illness and activity restrictions among women than men, figures that are matched by the numbers of men and women consulting a doctor. Of those inter-viewed for the General Household Survey in 2005, 11% of men and 16% of women said they had consulted an NHS GP in the 14 days prior to interview. While these figures are based on self-report and thus are to a certain extent unreliable, they do indicate a general trend that is supported by more objective measures of the presence or absence of illness in men and women.

The various risks that may explain the differences in morbidity and mortality can be divided into 'biological' (i.e. sex differences) and 'socio-cultural' (i.e. gender differences).

Biological risks linked to sex differences

Women	Men
Pregnancy and childbirth	Early onset heart disease
Breast cancer	Prostate cancer
Cervical cancer	
Menstrual irregularities	
Menopausal problems	

The list indicates some of the obvious sex differences between men and women that may influence morbidity and mortality. They are based on biological differences because their source lies primarily in the physiological differences between

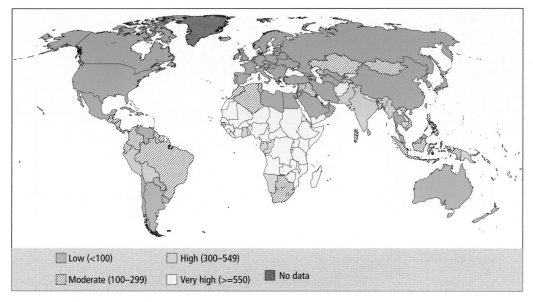

Low (<100) | High (300–549)
Moderate (100–299) | Very high (>=550) | No data

Figure 8.2 Maternal mortality ratio 2000 per 100,000 live births (Source: United Nations 2005).

men and women. However, the way in which these differences are responded to is dependent on society and the beliefs, values and attitudes of its members. For example, it is estimated that half a million women worldwide die each year as a direct consequence of pregnancy and childbirth, and more than 10 times that number are seriously disabled. Many of these problems occur in developing countries where health care services are not as accessible or affordable for women in difficulty before, during and after labour.

Figure 8.2 indicates where maternal mortality is particularly high: 95% of the world's maternal mortality occurs in Africa and Asia, with estimated death rates above 250,000 a year in each continent; in Latin America and the Caribbean the rates are less that one tenth of this (22,000); while in Europe, North America and Australasia they are one hundredth of this (2,500).

Morbidity statistics surrounding pregnancy and childbirth are even more telling than those for mortality.

Case study: prolapsed uterus in Nepal

Prolapsed uterus is a condition where the uterus comes through the vaginal opening due to the ligaments from the wall of the stomach being unable to support the organ. There are three degrees of prolapse:

1 The cervix appears at the vaginal opening when a woman is bearing down.
2 The cervix descends into the vulva.
3 The cervix and, in the most severe cases, the entire uterus extends beyond the vulva.

Lifting heavy objects, bearing many children, difficult confinements and giving birth to large babies all contribute to the likelihood of uterine prolapse. Heavy manual labour during pregnancy and malnourishment, both of which are the lot of many poor rural women, are likely to exacerbate the condition.

First and second degree prolapse often goes unrecognized by doctors, to whom poor rural women in Nepal have limited access, and embarrassment often prevents them seeking medical attention even where it is available. If detected early, a ring pessary is usually sufficient to keep the uterus in place. By the time a third degree prolapse develops, surgical removal is the only option, a treatment that is not affordable for the majority of rural women. Instead, they face a future of pain (particularly back and abdominal pain), ulcerous sores, profuse menstrual bleeding, urinary problems and a deteriorated sex life.

Figures for the incidence of uterine prolapse in Nepal are hard to calculate, but there are likely to be hundreds of thousands of sufferers representing a huge physiological and psychological burden on this developing country of 29 million people. Yet very little is being done to alleviate the problem. This compares with the US$400,000 spent on a single HIV/AIDS campaign in Nepal, where an estimated 58,000 people are HIV-positive.

Case study: prostate cancer – dying from embarrassment?

Cancer of the prostate is the second most common male cancer (after lung cancer) in Britain (Figure 8.3). Many men are unaware of where their prostate gland is and what it does. Fear and prudishness also conspire against men with prostate problems seeking advice and help. Compared to cervical cancer (which kills one tenth the number of women, mainly because of the effectiveness of the screening programme now available), there is no organized screening programme for prostate cancer in the UK. The two methods of screening – rectal examination and prostate-specific antigen (PSA) tests – are both unreliable and of limited help in diagnosing early disease, which is what is needed to save lives. Prostate cancer is a relatively slow-developing disease, although only a third of all new UK cases each year survive five years (the rate in the US is 65%). It is estimated that 80% of cases remain undiagnosed until the disease is advanced and prognosis is less good.

The musician Frank Zappa (d. 1994), French president François Mitterrand (d. 1996) and Jamaican president Michael Manley (d. 1997) all died of prostate cancer.

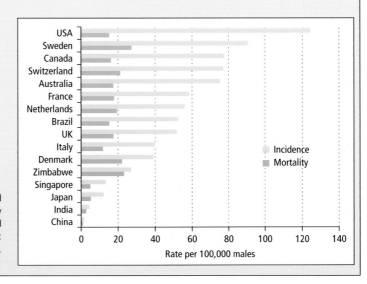

Figure 8.3 Age standardized (world) incidence and mortality rates, prostate cancer in selected countries, 2002 estimates (Source: Cancer Research UK: http://info. cancerresearchuk.org/cancerstats/).

Socio-cultural risks linked to gender differences

Women	Men
Infanticide	Alcohol/tobacco misuse
Rape	Accidents
Domestic violence	Suicide
Hormonal contraception	
Abortion	
Clitoridectomy	
Anorexia nervosa/bulimia	
Agoraphobia (85%)	
Anxiety and depression	

The list shows some of the risks linked to gender. They are socio-cultural rather than biological because their source lies primarily in the way society is organized and the beliefs, values, attitudes and (consequently) behaviours of individuals in society.

Case study: 'More than 100 million women are missing'

Figure 8.4 indicates the gender ratio between men and women in different countries around the world. The dark blue and light blue show the countries where the sex ratio of women to men is above 1.0; dark and light grey are the countries where this ratio is below 1.0; white represents countries either where there are no figures or where the difference in the gender ratio is insignificant. Some of the differences in gender ratios are due to labour migration between countries. However, a significant proportion is due to infanticide and unequal treatment of male and female children so that the survival rate to adulthood of boys is greater than that of girls (or, less commonly, vice versa). Socio-cultural factors such as the perceived need for male children to maintain the family name or high levels of dowry (bridewealth) required for girls to be able to marry are implicated.

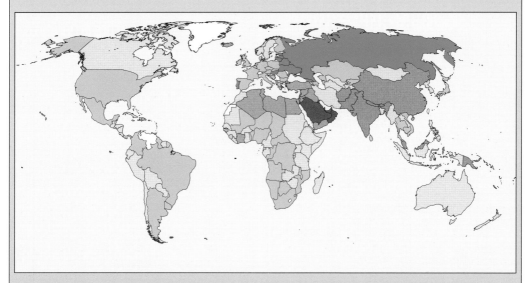

Figure 8.4 Gender ratio 2000 (Source: UC Atlas of Global Inequality: http://ucatlas.ucsc.edu/).

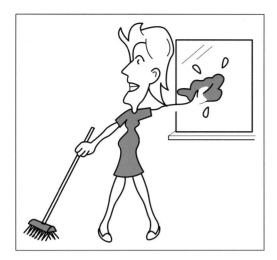

Figure 8.5 The 'second shift' of a working woman.

Inequalities of gender

The case of infanticide and unequal sex ratios is an extreme example of more general, gendered inequalities between men and women. It is fair to say that in no society do women enjoy the same opportunities as men. There are inequalities that have been identified in income, expectations of work and access to services, among others. These inequalities are supported by cultural ideas of what men and women should be like and how they should behave ('norms'), which in turn are the product of socialization.

The 'double burden' of working women

In many countries, both developed and developing, women's participation in the workforce is increasing. This is encouraging, since access to income has been identified as one of the main ways in which women can increase their household's means. However, this has not been matched by the increasing participation of men in household chores, leading to what is called the 'double burden' of women (or the 'second shift' – Figure 8.5).

> **Points of view: Norms, attitudes and beliefs about gender**
>
> Find a magazine or catalogue containing various images of men and women. What are your reactions to them? What do your reactions tell you about the norms and attitudes you hold, and the norms and attitudes of society?

The linking of sex and gender

It is not always possible to differentiate between the influence of the biological and the social in the different health experiences of men and women, as the next two case studies show.

> **Case study: Differential longevity with cystic fibrosis by sex and gender**
>
> Cystic fibrosis is the most common autosomal recessive gene disorder affecting Caucasians, with an incidence in the UK of about 1 in 2500. Through its effects on the exocrine system, which produces excessively thick mucus, it has serious consequences for the lungs, pancreas and digestive system, although with earlier screening and better treatment strategies, longevity has increased over the past few decades with many sufferers now surviving into adulthood. However, while the disease is not sex-linked and is fairly evenly distributed between males and females at birth, longevity differs markedly between men and women. In the UK, the median age of death from cystic fibrosis is currently over 30, but is two years higher for men than for women. In other parts of the world, this difference is even greater. In Australia, for example, the median survival rate for men is 41, whereas for young women it is 27.
>
> A study that took place with 40 young people suffering from cystic fibrosis in Victoria, Australia, in the late 1990s aimed to investigate the reasons for this discrepancy. Nineteen young men and 21 young women, roughly matched for the severity of their pulmonary disease, were interviewed. The study found that the experience of CF differed
>
> *(continued on p. 106)*

(continued)
according to gender. The greatest differences were in attitudes and approaches concerning the meaning of life, death, career, body image and treatment regime. There were significant differences associated with severity of the disease, but gender differences were also marked. The following statements from the young men (M) and young women (W) interviewed illustrate some of these.

Philosophy of life
'That's what I want to do . . . to be happy basically and to be happy and healthy.' (W, age 17)

'Living to the most you can, do everything you can possibly in life. To meet all your goals . . . live life through to 70'. (M, age 18)

[57% of women but only 21% of men expressed the likelihood that CF would affect their future]

Death
'. . . CF people don't really live much further than their twenties, late teens and I just always thought, oh well once I get to 21, 22, 23 I'll probably be dead . . . I mean there's not much of a life for people with CF.' (W, age 20)

    'I don't think about it much . . . it's too deep for me.' (M, age 17)

Career
'I was looking to more part-time work due to my CF . . . I'd need more time to physio and to keep my health, because I would have to put in so much at work and not wanting them to know I had CF.' (W, age 19)

'Some people choose their career around the fact that they've got CF, but I'm not bothering to. I'm just going to do what I do and see if I cope with it.' (M, age 19)

[17% of the men compared with 76% of the women took the disease into consideration in their career planning]

Body image
'Everyone wants to be strong, I think.' (M, age 18)

[For the young women, the thinness they had that was associated with the disease was seen as attractive; for the young men, it was something to be overcome by diet and exercise]

Treatment regimen
Exercise
'I hate sport . . . I've never been a sporty person, I just don't like it. No I'm not a sporty person which is hard.' (W, age 16)

[14% of women compared to 37% of men participated in exercise on a regular basis, and the exercise the young men took was generally more strenuous than that of the women]

Diet
[66% of women reported eating a low-calorie diet compared to 21% of men]

Physiotherapy
'I just didn't want to do it, I didn't see the point really.' (W, age 17)

[Thirty of the 40 young people interviewed did not carry out the suggested regimen; of these, 18 were women and 12 men. Seven out of nine who reported never following the suggested physiotherapy regimen were young women]

While the reasons for the differences in survival between men and women with cystic fibrosis are complex and include physiological ones (e.g. the average larger lung size of men), these gendered differences are striking and clearly play a significant part in the story.

Case study: Cardiovascular disease

Statements

1 Although the rates for women are lower than they are for men, CVD is still the leading cause of death for women in many industrialized countries.
2 Sex differences (e.g. the effects of oestrogen) affect the risk of developing CVD.
3 Gender differences affect the risk of developing CVD.
4 There are gender differentiated responses to CVD (among patients *and* health professionals).

Evidence for 1

Table 8.2 Age Standardised Mortality Rates from CVD in 1999 (35–74 year olds, per 100,000).

	Men	**Women**
Hungary	420	161
United Kingdom	249	89
USA	230	95
Finland	276	70
Japan	57	19

Source: World Health Organization (2003) www3.who.int/whosis

In the US in 2001:
- CVD was the leading cause of death for women (nearly 500,000 deaths annually).
- A woman was over 10 times more likely to die of CVD than of breast cancer.
- More women than men died of CVD (because of the ageing population).
- Mortality from CVD had decreased for men in the preceding 20 years, but not for women.

Evidence for 2

Table 8.3 Likely protective effects of oestrogen on the cardiovascular system.

Direct effects	Indirect effects
↑ Arterial vasodilation	↓ LDL-C
↑ Nitric oxide synthesis	↑ HDL-C
↑ Vasodilatory enzymes	↑ Triglycerides
↓ Vascular injury	↓ LDL-C oxidation
↑ Vascular endothelial cell growth	+ buffering stress responses?
↓ Vascular smooth muscle proliferation	

Evidence for 3

Some factors affecting the risk of developing CVD
Diet – in the UK women tend to eat more healthily than men.
Exercise – men and women tend to exercise differently.
Obesity – in almost all European countries, the prevalence of obesity is higher for women than for men, but men tend to develop more central or visceral fat, and central fat is more strongly correlated with CVD.

(continued on p. 108)

(continued)

Smoking – men are tending to give up smoking at a faster rate than women. (There are, however, significant ethnic differences in smoking that are gendered, see below.)

Stress – men and women have different experiences of stress. Women tend to occupy work roles that give them less control over the pace and nature of their work; in addition, they have the 'double burden' to contend with (see above).

Stress response – men and women have different responses to stress. Men are more likely to use alcohol as a coping mechanism for dealing with stress; men and women make largely similar reports of anxiety during the working week, however, urinary adrenaline samples (a physiological marker of stress) taken in the late afternoon tend to be higher in men than women.

Evidence for 4

Men's responses to heart attacks: the role of masculinity

A study conducted in 1991 found that men who scored higher on an index of masculinity delayed longer before seeking help after the first warning signs of a heart problem than those who scored lower. This was because:

- Some noticed symptoms but did not interpret them as a heart problem.
- Some noticed symptoms and did not act on them.
- Some did not notice symptoms at the time, but could remember them afterwards.

In addition to patients' and carers' responses to CVD, several studies conducted in the UK have found responses to CVD among health professionals differ according to the sex of the patient:

- In one study, GPs monitored and treated men with heart disease more intensively than women with heart disease.
- Women with suspected myocardial infarction received less specialist care in hospital.
- Women received fewer investigations and less treatment than men.

Race and ethnicity – what's the difference?

There are parallels in the relationship between race and ethnicity to that between sex and gender (above).

Race refers to the biological division of a species into groups based on the frequency with which certain hereditary traits appear among its members. *Ethnicity* refers to the social division of people into groups based on their identification with shared cultural characteristics. Markers of ethnicity may include:

- Language
- Food
- Religion
- Clothing
- Origins
- Myths and traditions
- Music and art

Humans are not particularly diverse genetically speaking – over 99% of our genetic make-up is common to all racial groups, and there is almost as much genetic variation within as between groups. There are clearly differences in physical characteristics between people of different ancestry. However, the relevance of these differences to their health status is debatable. Many people are impossible to ascribe to a racial group anyway. Thus the concept of 'race' is of limited use in everyday health care, although an exciting new area known as 'racial medicine' using latest findings in the field of pharmacogenetics may be about to change this.

Ethnicity is self-ascribed and people may differ in the significance they attach to the ethnic markers identified in their lives. Categories change and are dynamic, and people's identification with them is situational (i.e. dependent on the context within which they find themselves) rather than permanent. For example, some people of African origin who are born in the UK might perceive themselves as Black African; others might prefer to classify themselves as Black British. People from the Indian subcontinent might want to define themselves as, for example, Gujaratis or Punjabis; but in the 2001 Census they were only offered the options of 'Indian', 'Pakistani', 'Bangladeshi' or 'other Asian'. How ethnicity is defined will change over time (e.g. because of social and political attitudes). Some years ago, the term 'black' was unacceptable, whereas now it is used by the individuals belonging to this group. With increasing contact between peoples, intermixing and sharing of ethnic markers can occur. This is known as 'hybridity'. The distribution of ethnic groups in the UK according to the 2001 Census is shown in Table 8.4.

There is an inherent racism in the way ethnicity is categorized in Table 8.4, because there are many 'white' ethnic minority groups who are not included (e.g. the Irish, Portuguese, Polish, Ukrainian). The proportion of ethnic minorities in the total population is increasing, largely as a result of higher population growth among these groups. One third of the ethnic minority populations as a whole are below 16 years compared to one fifth of the majority, white population. In the 'mixed' group, 55% of the population are below 16 years, indicating that this group is likely to increase markedly in the future. At the same time, the number of 'ethnic elders' is increasing, albeit more slowly.

The geographical distribution of ethnic minorities is uneven. Ethnic minorities constitute 9% of the total population of England, but only 2% of Scotland and Wales; 48% of all ethnic minorities are found in London, where they comprise 29% of the population.

Ethnic differences in health and illness

The bulk of the health problems of ethnic minority groups in the UK are similar to those of the majority white population, and are linked to their

Table 8.4 UK population by ethnic group, April 2001 (Source: National Statistics website: www.statistics.gov.uk).

	Total population		Minority ethnic population
	Count	%	%
White	54153898	92.1	n/a
Mixed	677117	1.2	14.6
Asian or Asian British			
Indian	1053411	1.8	22.7
Pakistani	747285	1.3	16.1
Bangladeshi	283063	0.5	6.1
Other Asian	247664	0.4	5.3
Black or Black British			
Black Caribbean	565876	1.0	12.2
Black African	485277	0.8	10.5
Black Other	97585	0.2	2.1
Chinese	247403	0.4	5.3
Other	230615	0.4	5.0
All minority ethnic population	*4635296*	*7.9*	*100*
All population	58789194	100	n/a

socio-economic position rather than their 'racial' or ethnic background. Ethnic minority populations in general experience more unemployment and low paid work. Racial discrimination is a factor directly influencing mental health (and possibly hypertension), as well as employment, housing and education, all of which affect health.

Biological differences linked to ethnic differences

Certain diseases are more prevalent in certain populations according to their genetic history and the evolutionary forces (such as natural selection) that they have experienced.

Case study: Sickle cell anaemia and the haemoglobinopathies

Sickle cell anaemia is a genetic disorder found at high frequencies in certain parts of world (notably Africa) and at higher frequencies among particular racial groups (Black Africans). It is caused by an autosomal recessive gene and is inherited in most cases. Where it appears in its homozygotic form the disease is usually fatal. However, its heterozygotic form gives protective benefit against infection by the *falciparum* malaria parasite.

The disease is marked by abnormally shaped red blood cells caused by defective haemoglobin. These blood cells get stuck in the small blood vessels, causing blockages that deprive organs and tissues of oxygen. Incapacitating pain in the joints and elsewhere is the principal symptom, sometimes accompanied by fever. Because the sickle cells die much sooner than a normal red blood cell, severe anaemia is also common.

Other haemoglobinapathies include thalassaemia, which is prevalent in malarial parts of Mediterranean, Africa and New Guinea and among populations whose ancestry is in these areas. In thalassaemia, haemoglobin is structurally normal, but is not produced in sufficient quantities. G6PD deficiency is a condition where a certain enzyme is deficient and gives immunity against malaria.

Haemoglobinpathies and the health services
The following are measures that can be taken to ameliorate the effects of the haemoglobinpathies and extend the longevity of sufferers.
- Blood transfusions; pain relief; fluid therapy.
- Prophylactic oral antibiotics in early life.
- Hydroxyurea (the first effective drug treatment for adults with severe sickle cell anaemia, reducing the frequency of painful crises and acute chest syndrome and leading to fewer blood transfusions)
- Regular health maintenance.
- Education of patients and carers.
- Referral to relevant support organizations.

Although the prevalence of the haemoglobinopathies is similar to that of cystic fibrosis and haemophilia, representatives of black and minority ethnic groups are critical of service provision in this area. Although early diagnosis enables protective measures that can increase longevity and quality of life, obstacles to the improvement of care include poor knowledge among health professionals, socio-economic and educational disadvantage among the groups in which prevalence is highest, and institutional racism (see page 126).

Inherited conditions account for only a small proportion of the ill health of different ethnic groups, however. The 'big killers' such as cancer and heart disease are the key problems facing most minority ethnic groups. However, there are some differences in disease incidence which may be due to a combination of biological and social factors. One such disease is type 2 diabetes.

Case study: Type 2 diabetes among South Asian and African-Caribbean populations in the UK

The WHO has recognized a 'global epidemic in diabetes', but it is a disease which people from some cultures or races seem to be particularly prone to (Figure 8.6). The prevalence of diabetes and impaired glucose tolerance is much

---

higher in South Asian and African-Caribbean ethnic groups in the UK than in the general population. Moreover, mortality from heart disease is three times higher in South Asian patients with diabetes compared to white British patients with the disease. Many of the other complications of diabetes, such as end-stage renal disease, are also higher. Dietary factors, such as increased total calorie intake, a relative excess of saturated fats and reduction in fibre, as well as reduced levels of physical activity, are the main features of the 'obesogenic' environment typical of western societies. However, the impact of these lifestyle factors on obesity and diabetes appears to differ between ethnic groups, and while differences in uptake of these features may explain some of this variation, genetic factors may play a more determining role than has hitherto been recognized.

A study of beliefs about diabetes amongst 40 Bangladeshi immigrants in London indicated a rich mixture of overlap with and differences from the medical model. The importance of diet was recognized, including the danger of consuming too much sugar. However, two sorts of foodstuffs were identified: 'nourishing' and 'digestible'. Foods that were nourishing were strong and gave energy, such as white sugar, meat, butter, fat and spices, and were seen as crucial to the maintenance of health. However, those with diabetes were considered to need weaker foods such as boiled rich or cereals. Indigestible foods were those that were raw, baked or grilled; only fried foods were deemed digestible. Molasses (liquid brown sugar) was considered safe for people with diabetes to eat.

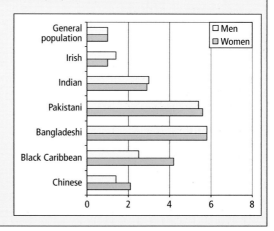

Figure 8.6 Prevalence of diabetes by ethnic group and sex, 1999, England, standardized risk ratios (Source: Health Survey for England: www.statistics.gov.uk).

Socio-cultural factors in ethnic differences affecting health

- Social support
- Alcohol and tobacco consumption
- Diet
- Beliefs about health, illness and the body
- Political and economic situation (e.g. being an asylum seeker)
- Access to and use of health and social care services

Social support

It is a stereotype to think that people from ethnic minorities necessarily come from large and close families. Where migrants come for work, it is frequently the men who travel, leaving families behind in their place of origin. The elderly similarly cannot be assumed to have good family support.

Alcohol and tobacco consumption

Minorities from the Indian subcontinent generally smoke and drink less than the UK general population (27% of the general population were reported to smoke in 1999), although there are exceptions, such as smoking rates among Bangladeshi men (44% in 1999), White Irish men and women (39%) and Black Caribbean men (35% in 1999). Women from all ethnic minority groups (except the White Irish who smoked at a higher rate than the general population) tended to smoke less than the average. Although very few Bangladeshi women smoked cigarettes, a relatively

111

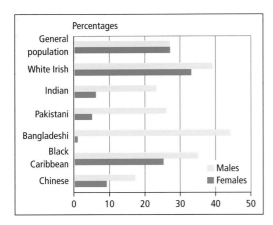

Figure 8.7 Cigarette smoking by ethnic group and sex, 1999, England (Source: Health Survey for England: www. statistics.gov.uk).

large proportion (26 per cent) chewed tobacco. This method of consuming tobacco was also popular among Bangladeshi men (19 per cent), but tended to be used in addition to cigarette smoking. Smoking behaviour is strongly related to socio-economic class, with people from lower socio-economic classes more likely to smoke than those from higher classes. The patterns of smoking in the different ethnic groups are partly explained by their socio-economic differences. For example, Bangladeshi men are over-represented in the lowest socio-economic class (semi-routine or routine occupations), and these men had the highest rates of smoking (see Figure 8.7).

Diet

There are significant differences among ethnic groups in terms of diet. Asians tend to eat less saturated fat and cholesterol and more polyun-saturated fat and vegetable fibre than the British population. This partly explains their low incidence of cancer of the bowel. However, it does not explain why the rate of CVD in this group should be so high.

Beliefs about health, illness and the body

Anthropologists have described many interesting variations concerning ideas about health, illness and the body in countries around the world, as well as the UK (see Chapter 2). These do not always translate into similar beliefs held by ethnic minority group members with ancestry from these countries in the UK. Considerable variation can exist within ethnic groups concerning these beliefs. For example, menstruation can be perceived as an opportunity to clear bad blood, or as a nuisance, and these perceptions may affect what kind of birth control is recommended to an individual woman. 'Hot' and 'cold' foods may be regarded as important in maintaining a balanced body. Some Muslim patients are characterized as having a fatalistic approach to their illness. However, invoking the operation of God's will is very much an idiom rather than implying that they believe there is nothing they can do to improve their health.

Access to and use of health services

People from ethnic minorities often have different ways of dealing with illness. There may be more use made of traditional remedies and practitioners (see Chapter 5). GP consultation rates tend to be higher among ethnic minority groups (excluding the Chinese) compared to the general population. A study conducted in 1999 found that the consultation rate (the percentage who consulted a GP in the past two weeks) for Bangladeshi men was 22%, and 15–17% for Indian, Pakistani and Black Caribbean men, compared to the general population (12%). The figures for women were broadly similar.

Steps to enhance health care among minority ethnic groups

- Patient profiling.
- Removing barriers to access through:
  - working with reception staff;
  - raising awareness of services and health issues;
  - improving physical access and appointment systems;
  - ensuring culturally acceptable provision.
- Enhancing effective communication through:

○ general principles of good communication;
○ negotiating language and cultural barriers.
• Developing local cultural knowledge.

• responding to the individual.
• awareness of attitudes – stereotyping, prejudice and racism.

Points of view: Bilingual support

Communication skills are applicable to all patient–professional interactions and involve non-verbal communication, courtesy, interest, respect and active listening, as well as imparting information clearly and effectively. However, language barriers are major obstacles, particularly for women and older people from South Asian and Chinese groups, refugees and asylum seekers.

What are the options in terms of bilingual support to overcome these barriers and what are the advantages and disadvantages of each? Some suggestions appear below.

Option	Comment
Defer the consultation until language assistance can be obtained	May be necessary where situation is not urgent
Use a trained interpreter, either in the consultation room or telephone-based using the website www.languageline.co.uk	Tend to be underused. May be expensive. Use varies considerably between general practices. Have received training specific for health care
Recruit bilingual staff	Can be done through local black and minority ethnic group language publications. Should be valued by paying appropriate salary
Learn elements of the local language	Time-consuming and dependent on linguistic skills of practitioner
Use friends or family to interpret	May be effective, but make more frequent errors than professional interpreters, including distorting the meaning of the interpreted language, and may impose their own agenda rather than that of the patient. Confidentiality issues. Using children is not acceptable

---

If using an interpreter, the following key points are helpful:
• Make sure seating arrangements are suitable.
• Speak directly to the patient.
• Be aware of non-verbal communication.
• Avoid jargon and idiomatic speech.

• Check the patient's understanding.
• Use written materials translated into the patient's own language.
• Despite the extra time taken, always ask patient at the end if there is anything they have not understood or wish to discuss.

Pharmacogenetics – a future for racial medicine?

Pharmacogenetics studies the extent to which genetic differences influence the response of individuals to medicines. We know there is considerable variation in this response among individuals due to age, sex, physiology and disease state, and because of interactions with other drugs. It is likely that every pathway of drug metabolism is affected by genetic variability. This variation is often related to the actions of drug metabolizing enzymes such as CYP2D6 (one of the cytochrome P-450 enzymes – a super-family of microsomal drug-metabolizing enzymes). Until recently, this

(continued on p. 114)

(continued)

variation was regarded as unimportant. However, recent research has found that individuals vary genetically in their CYP2D6 metabolism, from showing no function to greater than average function, with striking consequences for the pharmacokinetics and therapeutic effects of drugs metabolized by this enzyme, including:

- Tamoxifen (used in the treatment of breast cancer)
- Codeine (pain relief)
- Dextromethorphan (a cough suppressant)
- Metoprolol (a beta blocker)
- Nortriptyline (an anti-depressant)
- Debrisoquin (a hypertensive drug)

If the genetics of drug susceptibility were better understood, it would be possible to develop personalized drug treatments that would optimize the dose of any drug.

Adverse drug reactions (ADRs) are responsible for about 6.5% of acute hospital admissions. Meta-analysis of studies of ADRs has indicated the following risks resulting from treatment by drugs used in cardiovascular medicine by ethnic group:

Angio-oedema due to angiotensin converting enzymes (ACE) inhibitors
Black patients have a relative risk of 3.0 compared to non-black patients.

Cough due to ACE inhibitors
Chinese, Korean and Japanese patients have a relative risk of 2.7 compared to white patients.

Intracranial haemorrhage due to thrombolytic therapy
Black patients have a relative risk of 1.5 compared to non-black patients.

Moderate or severe bleeding after treatment with thrombolytic therapy
Black patients are at an increased risk of 1.9 compared to non-black patients.

If genetic markers for severe ADRs could be found, this would help identify patients at high risk before starting treatment.

BiDil

A recent development in the field of pharmacogenetics is research into a combination pill, BiDil, to treat heart failure among black Americans, who are $2\frac{1}{2}$ times more likely than whites to develop the disease. As well as the increased risk of ADRs, ACE inhibitors, the standard drugs for heart failure, were known not to work as well among black patients. Two chemicals – isosorbide dinitrate and hydralazine – taken in combination help boost the levels of nitric oxide (important for cardiac health) in the heart. Studies in the 1980s involving mostly white patients who were given the chemicals separately found they offered no benefit. However, the few black patients in the studies did seem to benefit, and so a trial of 1050 black patients was launched in June 2001. Half got standard heart failure drugs and a placebo; the other half got standard drugs plus BiDil. The decreased mortality in the group taking BiDil was so dramatic that the trial was halted after three years so that the placebo group could be switched to the drug in order to benefit from it too. After one year, only 6.2% of the patients given BiDil had died compared to 10.2% who were given the standard heart failure drugs. The rate of first heart failure hospitalization reduced from 24.4% to 16.4% among the BiDil users, and the quality of life score of those on BiDil improved from 2.7 to 5.6. However, there were some side-effects such as increased rates of headaches and dizziness.

Some people worry that although the drug might not be the best choice for every patient they will automatically be prescribed the 'black pill' solely on the basis of their skin colour. It is uncertain what the benefits will be for those of mixed race and whether it might be of benefit to whites (who were not offered it in combination). However, BiDil represents something of a watershed in the effort to develop medicines that can be targeted at specific racial groups and/or individuals in order to improve not only safety but also efficacy, in preference to the 'one medicine fits all' approach that has been characteristic of much medical practice to date.

Cultural competency

A little knowledge can be a dangerous thing!

Knowing that gender and ethnicity have a part to play in disease risk, the experience of disease and disease outcomes is better than ignorance. Knowing that CVD is a major killer of women as well as of men, for example, helps overcome the stereotype that CVD is a 'male' disease, and should ensure quicker response times and better treatment for women, who currently get a raw deal from the health services compared to men. However, a little knowledge can be a dangerous thing and may contribute to the development of new stereotypes as well as overcoming old ones.

'Cultural stereotyping' is reflected in the tendency to make statements of 'the "x" do this' type, where 'x' is an ethnic group, men, women, the elderly, young people or whoever. Stereotyping is a common psychological process in everyday life which enables us to make decisions more quickly. However, in medical practice it can be dangerous, since it makes assumptions about patients that may lead to quite inappropriate treatments. This has been observed in contraceptive provision, for example, where family planning practitioners decide that a woman a) needs contraception, and b) is best suited for a particular type of contraception, without first finding out whether she wants contraception and, if she does, offering her all the options so that she can make an informed decision for herself.

Doctors may meet someone from any cultural background and any ethnic group. And one can never know all the facets of every ethnic group or religion. Even if one could, knowing all there is to know about (say) Islam, or the genetic makeup of people from a specific country, one would still not be in a position to know whether the particular patient one was working with fitted the knowledge one had. Many members of a particular religious faith, for example, describe themselves as 'lapsed' or 'non-practising', and there are degrees of observance in people from all religious groups,

and many small but often significant differences between and within ethnicities, regions, families and individuals. Sensitivity to cultural difference provides a basis from which you can begin to ask well-informed questions about the needs of your patient.

This sensitivity to cultural difference leads to a greater level of *cultural competency*. This term encapsulates a number of elements:
- The capacity for cultural self-assessment, and the assessment of others, being mindful that everyone is an individual first and representative of a cultural group second
- Consciousness of the dynamics inherent when cultures interact
- The institutionalization of culture knowledge
- The adaptation of service delivery to reflect an understanding of cultural diversity.

Summary

- Sex is the biologically derived differences between men and women; gender is the socio-culturally derived difference.
- Women tend to suffer greater morbidity while men suffer earlier mortality. The reasons for this concern both biology and culture.
- Ideas about 'femininity' and 'masculinity' lead to inequalities between the sexes and contribute to the greater health burden of women.
- Race is the biologically derived difference between population groups; ethnicity is socio-culturally derived.
- Inherited conditions account for only a small proportion of the health inequalities of different ethnic groups.
- The 'big killer' diseases in the UK affect ethnic minority populations just as they do the majority population, although their distribution varies.
- There are relatively straightforward ways in which health care provision for ethnic minority groups can be enhanced.
- Pharmacogenetics promises greater drug efficacy and safety for individuals and racial groups.
- Stereotyping is a process that spans gender and ethnicity and can lead to inadequate and/or inappropriate treatment.

• Cultural competency is a means of overcoming stereotyping and valuing diversity.

Further reading

Greenhalgh, T., Helman, C. and Chowdhury, A. M. (1998) Health beliefs and folk models of diabetes in British Bangladeshis: a qualitative study. *British Medical Journal*, **316**: 978–83.

Helgeson, V. S. (1995) Masculity, men's roles, and coronary heart disease. In D. Sabo and D. F. Gordon (eds) *Men's Health and Illness*. Thousand Oaks, CA: Sage, pp. 68–104.

Kai, J. (ed.) (2003) *Ethnicity, Health, and Primary Care*. Oxford: Oxford University Press.

McDowell, S. E., Coleman, J. J. and Ferner, R. E. (2006) Systematic review and meta-analysis of ethnic differences in risks of adverse reactions to drugs used in cardiovascular medicine. *British Medical Journal*, **332**: 1177–80.

Mendelsohn, M. E. (2002) Protective effects of estrogen on the cardiovascular system. *American Journal of Cardiology*, **89(12)**, Suppl. 1: 12–17.

Sen, A. (1990) More than 100 million women are missing. *New York Review of Books* (20 December): 61–6.

Subba, B., Adhikari, D. and Bhattarai, T. (2003) The neglected case of the fallen womb. *Himal South Asia Magazine*, April. http://www.himalmag.com/2003/april/analysis.htm.

United Nations (2005) *The Millennium Development Goals 2005 Report*. New York: United Nations. See also http://www.un.org/docs/summit2005/MDGBook.pdf.

Willis, Miller, E., R. and Wyn, J. (2001) Gendered embodiment and survival for young people with cystic fibrosis. *Social Science and Medicine*, **53(9)**: 1163–74. See also http://www.cfww.org/pub/edition_1/Gender_and_Survival_for_Young_People_with_CF.asp.

Chapter 9

Mental health, illness and health care

Introduction

The problems of definitions and diagnosis common to all areas of medicine are probably at their most acute in the field of mental illness. Unlike physical conditions, which are usually expressed through physical symptoms and signs (i.e. what a patient has), mental illness is much more often expressed through behaviour and/or what is said (the patient's verbal and non-verbal communication). This leaves mental illness, and our understanding of its causes, diagnosis and treatment, very much more prone to the influences of culture and society, specifically to what is regarded as normal and abnormal communication in that society. This is reflected in the number of 'culture-bound syndromes' that can be identified – problems unique to a particular culture and society at a given point in time.

In any one year, 25% of the adult population in England are likely to experience some form of mental health problem; 30% of all GP consultations are for some kind of mental health condition, and 50–75% of GP consultations have a broadly psychiatric component. People with mental illnesses frequently experience problems in the way they think, feel or behave, which can significantly affect their relationships, work and quality of life. Mental illness causes problems not just for the individual, also but for his or her family, friends and carers. Apart from the incalculable burden of personal and family suffering, mental illness is estimated to cost the UK about £32 billion each year, including almost £12 billion in lost working days and approximately £8 billion in benefits payments.

There is much ignorance and fear surrounding mental illness. Those diagnosed may find themselves the subject of prejudice, stereotyping and discrimination which, with the other forms of social and economic disadvantage they encounter as a result of their illness, further exacerbate their problems. However, most people with mental illness can lead productive and fulfilling lives if given appropriate treatment and support, of which medical treatment may be only a small part. In order to discourage the medicalization of mental illness, the mental health charity MIND prefers to use the term 'mental distress' rather than 'mental illness'. While the term 'distress' emphasizes the pain of the patient, it does not reflect the relational aspects of mental illness – the effects on others, which is often the most salient concern of non-patients. 'Mental disorder' is another term sometimes used to evoke a less medicalized understanding of mental illness, but this has legal associations that are much broader than clinical diagnosis. In fact, the terms used to denote 'mind

Lecture Notes: *The Social Basis of Medicine*, 1st edition. By Andrew Russell. Published 2009 by Blackwell Publishing. ISBN: 978-1-4051-3912-0

problems' are something of a minefield and reflect the many different cultural frameworks for understanding the mind.

Psychiatry is becoming more 'evidence-based' in its practice, but there remains much controversy about the nature, causes and treatment of mental illness. Despite recent government initiatives, it is still something of a 'Cinderella' discipline: under-represented in medical curricula and training, and relatively poorly resourced. Fewer than half of GPs have postgraduate training in psychiatry and only 2% of practice nurses have mental health training, although about half of GP surgeries provide counselling.

Advances in genetics and neurology have raised the profile of mental illnesses which are more 'organic' in their causation (i.e. those that are demonstrably linked to some kind of physiological or anatomical abnormality). However, as befits what is by far the most complex organ of the human body, disturbances in the brain are the hardest to detect and typify. Brain scans and brain imaging have shifted the boundaries concerning clusters of symptoms that were previously distinguished as 'functional' psychoses (e.g. schizophrenia) and 'organic' ones (e.g. dementia). Future advances in this area may lead to further knowledge breakthroughs. However, understanding the social basis of mental health, illness and health care will remain crucial if doctors are to be effective not only in treating people with mental health problems or difficulties, but also in addressing the ways in which mental illness is thought about and categorized.

> ### This chapter covers the following topics
>
> Cultural theories of psychology and the mind
> The social context of normal and abnormal
> Socio-cultural influences on the diagnosis of mental illness
> Culture-bound syndromes
> Inequalities and mental illness
> Organization of mental health care services in the UK
> Legal dimensions of mental health care

Cultural theories of psychology and the mind

Mental health and mental illness are highly influenced by the culture and society in which an individual lives. Culture will influence that individual's ideas about psychology and the mind. The Cartesian dualism of much western thought separates 'mind' and 'body', leading to the sometimes unhelpful categorization of certain disorders as 'psychosomatic', which should not be interpreted as 'just psychological'. In other cultures, psychological and social disorders are patterned into mainly physical symptoms and signs, a process known as 'somatization'. Somatization is sometimes at work when depressed people present with diffuse, changeable and non-specific symptoms (e.g. 'tiredness', 'headaches', 'dizziness' and 'pains everywhere') although not everyone who presents with these symptoms is necessarily depressed.

Different cultures have their own understandings of psychology which affect ideas about the causation of mental disorder, its treatment and prognosis. In Chapter 2, we saw how explanations of ill health can be attributed to individual, natural, social and supernatural causes. What might be seen as the result of witchcraft in one society may be interpreted as spirit possession in another and as mental illness in a third. Even if we accept an interpretation of mental illness (or disorder), our models of its causation – and hence its treatment – will be influenced by dominant cultural values and assumptions. A good psychiatrist recognizes the majority of mental health problems as multifactorial in their aetiology, but a neurologist might look for an organic (i.e. biological) cause to remedy, a psychologist will be impressed by the 'learning history' of the individual and attempt to rectify that, and some 'radical psychiatrists' and social scientists may argue for the importance of social factors, i.e. that the cause of mental disorder is to be found in the family and/or society and must be dealt with at those levels.

The social context of normal and abnormal

Mental disorder derives from the inner, psychological state of an individual or group. In the absence of organic pathology, this state can only be indirectly appraised through observation and communication. Much of the basis for such an appraisal is how normal or abnormal the individual sufferer appears to be. Normality (or the lack of it) is interpreted on the basis of the tone and content of what people say, and non-verbal cues such as their dress, behaviour (e.g. posture, facial and body gestures), hairstyle, make-up and smell.

Many of these elements are quite context-specific. For example, a lecturer delivering a lecture to medical students in a lecture hall as part of a course in the social and behavioural sciences would generally be regarded as exhibiting 'normal' behaviour. Were he or she to do the same thing in a shopping centre, this behaviour would be regarded as 'abnormal' and would probably lead to instant referral to the local mental health care team. A child talking to himself, apparently in response to voices, is regarded as imaginative; such behaviour in an adult is regarded as evidence of schizophrenia. In some cases, abnormal behaviour is tolerated because it is associated with immense creativity – the 'mad genius' creating literature, art, music or engaged in other intellectual pursuits. Other examples of behaviour that would be regarded as indicative of pathology and a diagnosis of mental illness in some contexts yet are regarded as acceptable in others are outlined below.

The social context of mental health and illness – examples

Behaviour	Context and interpretation I	Context and interpretation II
Killing 'the enemy'	In wartime: a hero	In peacetime: a psychopath
Hearing voices telling you how to heal	In many Central and South Asian societies: a shaman – interlocutor between people and the spirit world	In western societies: a schizophrenic
Convulsions akin to epilepsy	Societies with a belief in the spirit world: possession, a state that is often respected and leads to a healer/oracle role	Societies without a belief in the spirit world: epilepsy, a stigmatized condition that, uncontrolled, can lead to abnormality

Some forms of abnormality in the examples above are acceptable in 'controlled' situations (e.g. wartime; during certain healing rituals) but not at other times. Historical context also plays a part. Joan of Arc was a French peasant girl in the fifteenth century who, directed by the voices of saints, changed the political history of France and was canonized by the Roman Catholic Church in 1920. By modern psychiatric diagnosis she would almost certainly have been regarded as schizophrenic.

There are many examples of opportunities for controlled abnormality at certain times of year. For example, at Hogmanay (New Year celebrations in parts of Scotland) and Mardi Gras (Shrove Tuesday carnival in parts of the Caribbean and South America), people may legitimately engage in behaviour which would be totally unacceptable at other times. Only when abnormal behaviour is uncontrolled or uncontrollable is it sometimes taken to be 'mental illness'. Again, societies differ in their tolerance of such abnormality and what constitutes it. In the former Soviet Union, the actions of political dissidents were deliberately labelled as mental abnormality ('sluggish schizophrenia') and many were compulsorily detained in psychiatric institutions as a result.

Statistically-based measures of 'normality' or 'abnormality' are inadequate as a means of determining mental health status. Statistically speaking, happiness is probably abnormal, but is not regarded as an undesirable mental state. Nor is a mental state that can be associated with mental disorder always undesirable. Anxiety, for example, does not necessarily involve problem behaviour and in certain contexts and to certain degrees (e.g. before exams) may be desirable as a means of improving performance. What is involved in determining 'caseness' (i.e. the point when a person becomes a patient with a 'case' of some kind of psychiatric complaint) in psychiatry are judgements based on the values and rules that govern behaviour in a given society.

Socio-cultural influences on the diagnosis of mental illness

Descriptions of madness have existed for several millennia, but it was only in the second half of the twentieth century that a number of increasingly fine-grained classificatory systems and diagnostic instruments for mental illness came into being.

Reasons for the development of classificatory systems and diagnostic instruments for mental illness

- Growth of epidemiology and its interest in classifying people as 'those with' and 'those without' disease, so that they can be counted.
- Government bureaucratic needs for numbers for policy and planning purposes (e.g. hospital provision). '
- The low degree of reliability between psychiatrists.
- The large numbers of troops exhibiting signs of mental distress during and after the First and Second World Wars who appeared to respond to treatment after short-term stays in institutions.

Epidemiology is relatively unproblematic in the case of physical ailments like bone fractures (where a 'yes/no' distinction is normally sufficient) or when there is a strong belief in the genetic and constitutional basis of mental illness, which was a feature of much psychiatric thinking until the 1940s. However, such an approach is less easily

squared with psychiatric concepts of 'overload', where the assumption is that everyone has elements of nervous illness in their psyche, but these only turn into illnesses when they exceed a certain level (i.e. a point on a scale), often due to psychosocial changes. Ascertaining whether a patient has reached a certain point is not unique to psychiatry, since much physical medicine also depends on setting a 'cut-off' point (e.g. for fever or for blood sugar levels). However, it is more problematic in psychiatry when the scales used are based on less tangible behavioural and expressed emotional features that serve to 'push the scale' or 'tip the balance' of an individual into 'caseness'.

The Diagnostic and Statistical Manual of Mental Disorders (DSM-I) was first developed in 1952 in the US with the intention of standardizing and formalizing the professional labelling of mental illness. It had a biopsychosocial focus, assuming that mental illness is the result of reactions to biological, psychological and social factors. In line with the 'overload' model, mental illnesses were not regarded as discrete, but as situated somewhere on a spectrum from normal to severe. DSM-II and DSM-III (published in 1968 and 1980 respectively) shifted the diagnostic criteria from a biopsychosocial to a disease model, based on descriptive patterns of symptoms rather than their aetiology, and an assumption that brain abnormalities caused mental illness. Such an approach was supported by the dramatic developments in knowledge of how the brain functioned and the ability of new generation pharmaceuticals to influence psychotic and neurotic symptoms, which suggested that neurobiology would provide all the answers. Homosexuality as a diagnostic category was dropped from DSM-III as a result of social and political pressure from the gay rights movement, and is a good example of how the diagnostic system is modified over time through shifts in socially derived views of acceptable behaviour and tolerance rather than exclusively by advances in scientific research. DSM-IV (1994) represents a shift back towards a more 'plastic' view of the brain, accepting that mood can change the biochemistry of the brain as well as vice versa.

The core psychiatric assessment

Core history
 Reason for referral
 Presenting complaint(s), and their history
 Psychiatric and medical history
 Alcohol and drug use

Core mental state examination (MSE)
 Appearance and behaviour
 Mood
 Speech
 Thoughts
 Perceptions
 Cognition
 Insight

Psychiatric classifications

Organic disorder, e.g. dementia, delirium
Learning disability, e.g. Down syndrome, autism
Substance misuse, e.g. alcoholism, opiate dependency
Psychosis, e.g. schizophrenia, bipolar disorder
Mood disorders, e.g. depression
Neurosis. e.g. anxiety disorders
Somatoform disorders, e.g. somatization disorder
Personality disorder, e.g. dissocial, histrionic
 personality
No psychiatric disorder

The other major classificatory system is the World Health Organization (WHO)'s International Classification of Diseases, 10th revision (ICD-10). While the two systems – DSM and ICD – are broadly similar, the ICD offers fewer major classification categories (e.g. no category for abnormal gender identity). Diagnoses based on either of the classification systems differ in their reliability (i.e. the extent to which psychiatrists agree on a patient's diagnosis). For example, the reliability for bulimia nervosa is relatively high, while for panic disorder it is low.

The validity of the classification systems (i.e. whether they measure what they claim to measure – the reality of the diagnostic categories themselves) is highly dependent on the reliability of the diagnosis and can be problematic in its own right. There are often major clinical differences between those diagnosed with the same disorder, for example in aetiology (cause), presentation (because of frequent comorbidities), the course of the illness and the outcome of treatment. Differences in the clinical criteria used in the diagnosis of particular conditions contribute to different rates of diagnosis in the UK and the US. For example, in the 1960s the diagnosis rates for schizophrenia in admission statistics to state mental hospitals in New York were five times those in the London. This prompted the US/UK diagnostic project which aimed to differentiate between cultural differences in diagnostic outcomes and to develop standardized measures of psychological abnormality across cultures. It found that when typical cases were presented (via video-taped interviews), concordance was high between psychiatrists on both sides of the Atlantic, but when 'mixed' cases were presented, American psychiatrists had a broader definition of schizophrenia and British psychiatrists a broader definition of bipolar affective disorder (also known as manic depression) which affected their diagnoses.

Case study: Factors affecting the psychiatric diagnosis – the power of peer influence

A US study conducted in the 1960s showed how likely practitioners were to follow the suggestions of assumed experts in reaching their diagnoses. Three groups of psychiatrists and clinical psychologists were shown the same video of an interview with an actor who had been trained to act out 'normal' behaviour and were asked to diagnose the patient's condition. The video the first group saw was prefaced with a high-prestige voice saying the patient looked neurotic but was actually psychotic. The second group were told the patient was entirely healthy. The third group received no voiceover. Results from this study were as follows:

(continued on p. 122)

(Continued)

Diagnosis	Neurosis/personality disorder	Psychosis	Normal
First group (N = 95)	63%	28.5%	8.5%
Second group (N = 20)	0%	0%	100%
Third group (N = 21)	43%	0%	57%

Case study: Factors affecting the psychiatric diagnosis – the power of labelling

A famous study published in 1973 involved eight actors undergoing diagnosis by psychiatrists in 12 different psychiatric hospitals. Each actor called a hospital for an appointment and arrived complaining they had been hearing voices that were 'empty', 'hollow' and 'unclear'. All other information, apart from the actor's occupation, was kept as close to the truth as possible. All eight actors were admitted, seven with a diagnosis of schizophrenia, and were able to go on to study life on the wards.

What this study may have shown is simply the cautiousness of psychiatrists (like all doctors) not to miss a 'real' problem, leading to many 'type II' errors (i.e. false positive diagnoses – classifying a healthy person as sick) rather than 'type I' errors (i.e. false negatives – classifying a sick person as healthy). A second study was carried out in which staff inducted into the study were told that stooges would in due course be trying to gain entry onto the ward. Forty-one cases of 'stooges' were diagnosed, even though no stooges were sent. Since then, the DSM-IV criteria have been tightened up so that a wider range of symptoms have to be present, for a longer period, in order for schizophrenia to be diagnosed than was previously the case. However, the risk of 'type II' errors remains high.

Individual experience and social stigma

A diagnosis can relieve a distressed person by labelling what is wrong. However, once a diagnosis is made, it can become a damaging label that is hard to shake off. For example, in western societies someone who has schizophrenia may come to be seen (and see themselves) as 'a schizophrenic' and little else. Moreover the concern with establishing a diagnosis may also do a disservice to the patient's experience of 'their' illness, which may have many more facets and meanings for them than can be encompassed purely by a diagnostic label.

Case study: 'Every Family in the Land' – changing minds

The Royal College of Psychiatrists set up a five-year campaign in 1998 to increase the understanding of mental health problems and reduce their stigma. It aimed to increase understanding of six common mental disorders: alcohol and other drug misuse, anxiety, anorexia nervosa and bulimia, depression, Alzheimer's disease and dementia, and schizophrenia. It intended to challenge preconceptions about them, and to close the gap between what health professionals and the public perceive as useful treatments.

Ways for health professionals to challenge the stigma of mental disorder include the following:
- Examine one's own attitudes.
- Update one's knowledge of mental illness.
- Listen to what patients say about mental illness and its consequences.
- Watch out for and challenge stigmatizing language (e.g. 'someone with schizophrenia' rather than 'a schizophrenic' or 'a nutter').
- Be an advocate for those with mental illness.
- Challenge stigma in the media through letters and emails.

Culture-bound syndromes

Culture-bound syndromes (also called culturally specific syndromes) are a group of disorders which are unique to a particular group of people, culture or geographical area. They are referred to in DSM-IV as 'locality-specific patterns of aberrant [deviant] behaviour and troubling experience that may or may not be linked to a particular DSM-IV diagnostic category'. This definition reflects the differences in opinion that exist as to whether these syndromes are different cultural manifestations of underlying psychiatric problems that are universal, or whether they are psychiatric problems that are truly unique to a particular group. Most are reactive disorders of some sort.

Some examples of culture-bound syndromes

Hikikomori

Hikikomori is a Japanese term for acute social withdrawal and is a condition that has been the subject of considerable media attention in Japan over the last few years. It mainly affects middle-class young men who seem otherwise in good health. They withdraw completely from society by locking themselves in their rooms for extended periods – one man was found to have remained in his room for over 20 years. There have been a few high-profile cases where young men have emerged from their homes and committed violent crimes, including murder. However, it is wrong to call *hikikomori* the homicidal disease because most sufferers tend towards depression and lethargy rather than violence. It is also associated with agoraphobia, insomnia and obsessive-compulsive disorders. Sufferers also often have persecution complexes and may exhibit regressive behaviour. The Japanese government considers *hikikomori* to be a social rather than a mental disorder. Sometimes it is triggered by bullying or excessive pressure to perform. As families sometimes collude in the withdrawal and hide the evidence from neighbours and friends, it is difficult to ascertain how many people are affected, but realistic estimates put the figure at several thousand.

Arctic hysteria

There are various conditions among the indigenous inhabitants of the North American circumpolar regions associated with nutritional deficiencies and cultural beliefs. Among the Inuit of northern Canada, *pibloqtoq* is a condition whereby the sufferer becomes withdrawn and irritable, and may subsequently run outside stripping off all his or her clothes. They may end up having a convulsion, and upon waking appear calm and normal again. *Pibloqtoq* may be associated with dietary deficiency; it has been hypothesized that a shortage of calcium in the diet may precipitate an attack. Among the Algonquian Indian communities in Alaska and northern Canada a similar hysteria was reported by early explorers with a more elaborate form, based on beliefs in the *windigo* (*wendigo*, *witiko*), a malevolent, flesh-eating spirit. *Windigo* psychosis was described as a condition whereby the sufferer became not only violent but also obsessed with the notion of eating human flesh. Cases were mostly dealt with through curing rituals enacted by traditional healers (which often involved eating hot fatty meat) and in the rare event of these failing the sufferer might request to be executed before he could cause harm. The condition was particularly prevalent towards the end of the winter when food supplies were at their lowest and was believed to be likely if an individual had ever resorted to cannibalism during periods of famine in the past. Hence belief in the *windigo* could be seen as a powerful deterrent to cannibalism in these circumstances. Recently, researchers have queried whether *windigo*, always rare and of largely historical interest, was actually based on a misunderstanding by early explorers of a traditional myth.

Anorexia nervosa

Anorexia nervosa is an eating disorder in which the patient avoids eating or eats extremely little out of a fear of being or becoming fat. The condition is most common in young women between the ages of 12 and 21, but is not unknown among men (e.g. athletes and dancers) and older women. The fear/perception of being fat does not diminish as the individual loses weight, which they may do to an often dangerous and life-threatening extent. Both anorexia nervosa and bulimia (excessive eating followed by self-induced vomiting and/or purging with laxatives) are believed to be specific to western societies. In the Pacific islands, for example, such conditions or their equivalents are virtually unknown. Anorexia nervosa is associated with people who are comparatively wealthy for whom food is readily available and relatively abundant. It is also strongly associated with cultures in which 'thin is beautiful' and has been interpreted as the desire to be in control among those who feel powerless and for whom food denial is a means of reclaiming control over the self.

Points of view

Discuss the following conditions as possible examples of western 'culture-bound syndromes':
 Gulf War syndrome
 Deliberate self-harm
 Agoraphobia (fear of open or public spaces)
 Road rage

Inequalities and mental illness

Table 9.1 is based on a nationwide survey using face-to-face interviews with adults aged 16–74. It shows that mood and neurotic disorders are much more common than functional psychoses such as schizophrenia – 12% had consulted their GP with some kind of mental health, nervous or emotional problem during the preceding 12 months; and 17% of those in social classes IV and V reported having consulted compared to 8% in social classes I and II.

Gender and mental illness

The psychoses are fairly evenly divided between men and women. However, the neurotic and mood disorders (except panic disorder) are all significantly more numerous among women. Agoraphobia, for example, has a male:female distribution ratio of approximately 1:15. Behavioural problems such as drug and alcohol dependence are more commonly found among men. Suicide is also more common among men (see Chapter 11).

Table 9.1 Prevalence of psychiatric disorders: Great Britain, 2000 (adults age 16–74).

	All	Females	Males
Rates per 1000 population in the past week			
Mixed anxiety/depressive disorder	88	108	68
Generalized anxiety disorder	44	46	43
Depressive episode	26	28	24
Obsessive-compulsive disorder	11	13	9
Panic disorder	7	7	7
All phobias	18	22	13
All neurotic disorders	164	194	135
Rates per 1000 in past year			
Functional psychoses	5	5	6
Alcohol dependence	81	32	130
Drug dependence	37	21	54

Note: Some people may appear in more than one category.
Source: Psychiatric Morbidity Survey, National Statistics: www.statistics.gov.uk

Case study: Why are women more prone to depression?

Research has shown that depression in both men and women is typically provoked by severe threatening life events. However, it is anything up to twice as common among women as among men. Researchers seeking to understand the reasons for this difference studied 100 couples who had all experienced a serious life event that could be expected to provoke depression. Of these 56% of women and 40% of men had experienced depressed mood, of whom two-thirds of the women and half the men reported symptoms indicating clinical depression. Investigators were interested in whether the differences could be explained through artefact (e.g. women over-reporting mild forms of distress or men underplaying the severity of past episodes). However, by categorizing the different symptoms, they were able to discount this possibility. There was speculation that men develop alternative disorders in response to stress, such as alcohol abuse or antisocial behaviour, rather than depression. However, no increased incidence of alcohol or drug abuse was found in this group as a response to the life event, and more women than men reported feelings of anger in response to the crisis. Finally, the hypothesis that biological factors such as hormonal changes with pregnancy and childbirth might be important was discounted since there were no significant differences in depression scores between women who had given birth and those who had not.

The researchers concluded that the higher risk of depression following a crisis was due to gender differences in roles and the stresses and expectations that went with them, leading to different experiences of life events. Crises involving money, work or marital relationships had the same effect on both men and women in couples. However, following crises concerning children, housing and reproduction, women's risk of depression was more than five times that of men facing the same situation. The researchers found that women were more likely to hold themselves responsible for such events, while men were more likely to distance themselves from them.

Ethnicity and mental illness

Ethnic monitoring of publicly funded mental health services became mandatory in 1995. One in five mental health in-patients comes from a black or minority ethnic (BME) background, compared to about one in ten of the population as a whole. Research indicates that incidence rates for psychotic disorders among African Caribbean people are 2–8 times higher than among the white population. Some groups – notably black Caribbean, black African and other black groups – are more likely to have been detained under the Mental Health Act 1983 (see below), and are over-represented in psychiatric hospitals.

The 2001 Census showed that men from black and white/black mixed groups had rates of admission to psychiatric hospitals that were three times higher than the general population, while white British, Chinese and Indian men were less likely than the average population to be admitted. These figures were supported by a survey carried out on one day in 2006 of 32,023 in-patients on mental health wards in 238 NHS and private hospitals. The survey found that 21% of patients were from black and minority ethnic groups, although they represent only 7% of the population. Rates of admission were lower than average in the white British, Indian and Chinese groups, but three or more times higher than average in black African, black Caribbean and white/black Caribbean mixed groups. People in these three groups were more likely to be admitted to hospital, and were 19–39% more likely to have been admitted involuntarily. Once in hospital, black Caribbeans had the longest stay. These facts all point to elements of what has been termed institutional racism in the way black people with mental health problems are dealt with in the NHS and associated institutions (e.g. by the police and educational establishments). Some have suggested that the focus on schizophrenia is a racist obsession which overlooks other indicators that are better in the black Caribbean population than the general population, such as alcoholism.

Definition of institutional racism

The collective failure of an organization to provide an appropriate and professional service to people because of their colour, culture, or ethnic origin. This can be seen or detected in processes, attitudes, and behaviour that amount to discrimination through unwitting prejudice, ignorance, thoughtlessness, and racist stereotyping which disadvantages people in ethnic minority groups.

(Source: McKenzie and Bhui 2007)

Possible explanations for the high rates of schizophrenia amongst black Caribbean people include:

- Genetic factors
- Pregnancy and birth complications
- Social factors
    Social inequality
    Economic factors
    Discrimination
    Migration

- Racism
    Harassment
    Racial life events
- Demographic factors
    Density
    Age structure (predominantly young people)
    Numerator/denominator problems (e.g. young men avoiding Census-taking)
    Mobility.

Irish-born people living in the UK also have higher rates of mental disorder than the general population, including a higher rate of suicide than any other minority ethnic group. Studies suggest that psychological vulnerability to distress derives from previous experience in Ireland exacerbated by subsequent adverse social circumstances, life events and lifestyles following their arrival. High levels of alcohol consumption, social and familial disintegration, and depression seem to be linked among some members of this population.

Case study: 'Delivering Race Equality in Mental Health Care'

In January 2005, the Department of Health published a five-year action plan, 'Delivering Race Equality in Mental Health Care' (DRE). DRE aims to help English mental health services provide care that fully meets the needs of black and minority ethnic group patients and build stronger links with diverse communities.

The programme is based on three elements:

1 Providing more appropriate and responsive services and improving clinical services for specific groups, such as older people, asylum seekers, refugees and children

2 Engaging communities in planning services, supported by 500 new community development workers (CDWs)

3 Improving ethnicity monitoring, dissemination of information and knowledge about effective service, including a regular census of mental health patients

The vision for DRE is that by 2010 there will be: a service characterized by 'less fear' among BME communities and service users; increased satisfaction with services; a reduced rate of admission of people from BME communities to psychiatric in-patient units; a reduction in the disproportionate rates of compulsory detention of BME service users in inpatient units and a more balanced range of culturally appropriate and effective therapies.

Psychiatric disorders among the disabled

There is evidence that people with disabilities are more likely to suffer from mental health problems, or be labelled as having them, than the normal population. One indicative statistic is that profoundly deaf people are four times more likely than hearing people to be diagnosed as psychotic at some time in their lives.

Emotional and behavioural disorders are also more common in children and adults with learning disabilities than in the general population. Specific psychiatric disorders such as schizophrenia and biploar affective disorder are also more common. Various reasons help explain why:

- The organic cause of a learning disability may predispose to another psychiatric disorder (e.g. Alzheimer's disease in Down's syndrome).
- Communication problems, e.g. inability to express feelings after bereavement, which may lead to depression/anxiety.
- Higher rates of social deprivation, especially among those with mild learning disabilities.
- Vulnerability to abuse.
- Low self-esteem due to stigma/dependence on others.
- Frequent multiple losses – e.g. if living with parents until their deaths, may experience change of carer and home at the same time.

Organization of mental health care services in the UK

Mental health care in the UK is provided as part of both primary and secondary care. In England, 43 specialist mental health trusts provide acute inpatient care, community and rehabilitation services, residential care centres, day hospitals and drop-in centres. About 80,000 staff are employed in mental health services. The proportion of the NHS budget notionally intended for mental health services in 2004 was 15.9%, of which 80% went on inpatient services. Psychiatric hospital services have been progressively scaled down over the past 30 years through a process known as deinstitutionalization, whereby many services once provided by hospitals are now delivered in the community. Between 1996 and 2005 the number of beds available for acute mental health services in England was reduced by more than 20% (to 29,802), a trend which is continuing.

Factors encouraging deinstitutionalization

- Critical realization that those in asylums or other large institutions become 'institutionalized' and hence less capable functioning effectively outside.
- The development of new anti-psychotic medications enabling people to function in community settings.
- Cost savings of community care.
- Increasing concern for patient rights.

In the UK, 90% of people receiving help for mental health problems are dealt with in primary care. GPs now receive a financial incentive to provide for the physical health care needs of people with severe mental illness. Mental health care delivery is usually divided among a variety of general and more specialist mental health teams arranged on the basis of diagnostic categories and age.

Members of a typical Community Mental Health Team (CMHT)

Community psychiatric nurses
Social workers
Psychologists
Occupational therapists
Psychiatrists
Support workers
Manager

The titles, structure and functions of the teams represented in Figure 9.1 (see page 128) vary regionally and are continually changing. They are sometimes based on evidence of 'what works' in the field, and are sometimes a response to highly publicized failings in the system. For example, in 1992 Christopher Clunis, a known paranoid schizophrenia sufferer, stabbed a musician, Jonathan Zito, to death in a London underground station. This case prompted the establishment of assertive outreach teams to work with those severely ill patients who are reluctant to engage with the system.

According to the National Service Framework for mental health published in 1999, everyone seen by specialist mental health services should have their need for treatment assessed, a care plan drawn up and be assigned a named mental health worker to coordinate their care, including a regular review of their needs.

Legal dimensions of mental health care

The Mental Health Act 1983

There are two ways for a patient to enter a psychiatric unit. 'Informal admission' is when the patient

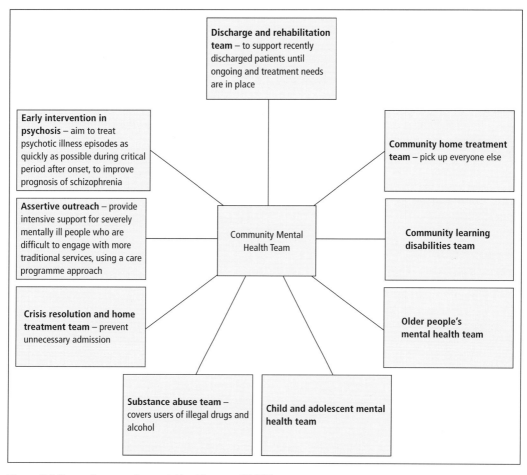

Figure 9.1 Types of community mental health teams (CMHT).

agrees, or does not object, to admission. They can discharge themselves at any time. However, one of the distinguishing features of mental health care that sets it apart from all other aspects of health care is that in some cases a person may be compelled to enter a psychiatric unit and receive treatment for their mental disorder. This is known as 'formal admission', and the measures by which this happens are contained in the Mental Health Act 1983. The Act applies to England and Wales; somewhat different rules apply in Scotland. The Act is complex; the sections most commonly used

to detain people (or 'section' them) are shown in the Table 9.2.

Table 9.2 shows the main kinds of 'civil admissions', i.e. the 94% of 27,400 formal admissions in 2005–6 of people not involved in criminal proceedings. Another 20,000 previously informally admitted patients were detained pending further assessment (by a doctor in charge, for a maximum of 72 hours). The proportion of formal admissions is increasing as the number of hospital admissions decreases. It was 18.7% of the total in 1994–5 and 27% of the total in 2003–4.

Table 9.2 Most commonly used routes of 'formal admission' to psychiatric units.

Act section	Type of admission	Maximum length of admission	Application	Criteria	Discharge
2	For assessment	28 days	Approved social worker (ASW) or nearest relative who has seen patient in previous 14 days, confirmed by two doctors	(a) Mental disorder warranting detention in hospital for assessment; and (b) It is in the interests of patient's own health or safety, or for the protection of others	Responsible medical officer (RMO), hospital managers, the nearest relative, who must give 72 hours' notice (the RMO can prevent her or him discharging a patient by making a report to the hospital managers) Mental Health Review Tribunal (MHRT). By patient applying within the first 14 days of detention
3	For treatment	Six months	ASW or nearest relative, confirmed by two doctors	(a) Patient suffering from mental disorder appropriate for medical treatment in hospital; and (b) such treatment is likely to 'alleviate or prevent a deterioration' of her or his condition; and (c) it is in the interests of patient's own health or safety, or for the protection of others that patient receives such treatment which cannot be provided unless she or he is detained	As above
4	For emergency admission	72 hours	ASW or nearest relative who has seen patient in previous 24 hours, confirmed by one doctor	(a) 'Urgent necessity' for the patient to be admitted and detained; and (b) waiting for a second doctor to confirm the need for an admission would cause 'undesirable delay'.	

Mental Capacity Act 2005

The Mental Capacity Act 2005 came into force in England and Wales in 2007. 'Mental capacity' means the ability of individuals to make decisions or to take actions that influence their life. An individual who has mental capacity should be able to:

- Understand information given to them to make a particular decision.
- Retain that information long enough to be able to make the decision.
- Use or weigh up the information to make the decision.
- Communicate their decision.

The Act makes it illegal to label someone 'incapable' merely because of their age, appearance, behaviour or medical condition/diagnosis. The Act aims to empower and protect people who are not able to make their own decisions some or all of the time. It also enables people to plan ahead for times when they may lose capacity through the provision of a lasting power of attorney (LPA) to appoint someone to make health, welfare and financial decisions on their behalf.

It can apply to both major decisions such as personal finance, medical treatment or where to live, or more everyday decisions, such as what to eat or wear. For everyday decisions, a relative or carer is the person most likely to assess capacity to make a particular decision, while professionals such as doctors or solicitors are more likely to assess capacity when decisions are more complex. Certain types of decision can never be made by another person, irrespective of mental capacity: these include marriage or civil partnership, divorce, sexual relationships, adoption and voting. The Act enables an individual to make an 'advance decision to refuse treatment' if there is a particular treatment they would not want if they ever lacked the capacity to refuse it. These advance decisions are legally binding and must be followed by doctors. On the other hand, advance decisions or consent do not apply to compulsory detention or treatment for a mental disorder under the Mental Health Act, whether or not someone has capacity.

The Mental Capacity Act applies to anyone aged over 16 in England and Wales, although in practice the majority of capacity issues are found in people over 50, such as the 750,000 people with dementia in the UK. It also protects people with other mental health problems, learning disabilities, stroke or brain injury. The Act sets out what happens when people are unable to make a particular decision, and makes it a criminal offence to ill treat or wilfully neglect a person who lacks capacity; on conviction there is a maximum term of imprisonment of five years.

The Act is based on five principles:

1 *Presumption of capacity* – that every adult has the right to make his or her own decisions and is assumed to have that capacity to do so unless it is proved otherwise. Capacity needs to be assessed for each new proposed procedure. For example, a person with learning difficulties (see Chapter 10) may have capacity to consent to a chest examination, but not to surgery for bowel carcinoma (due to their inability to understand the nature and likely outcomes of the more complex intervention).

2 *Maximizing decision-making capacity* – that all appropriate help and support should be provided before anyone concludes that an individual lacks capacity. If a person does not have the capacity and is unable to consent to a plan of treatment, then no one else can give or withhold consent on the incompetent person's behalf.

3 *Right to make eccentric or unwise decisions* – in other people's opinion.

4 *Best interests* – that anything done for a person who lacks capacity (e.g. if they are unconscious) must be in their best interests. This requires widespread consultation on the part of the doctor, including getting the views of family, carers, advocates and other professionals involved.

5 *Least restrictive intervention* – that anything done for a person without capacity must minimize restriction or curtailment of their basic rights and freedoms.

Practical provisions for the protection of vulnerable people are enshrined in the Act:

- A Court of Protection, which is able to make the final decision about whether someone lacks capacity, can make important decisions on someone's behalf, and can appoint deputies to make decisions on their behalf.

• An Office of the Public Guardian, which oversees Lasting Power of Attorneys, supports the Court of Protection, supervises Court-appointed deputies and gives guidance on the Mental Capacity Act to the general public.

• An Independent Mental Capacity Advocate (IMCA), who represents a person who lacks capacity but has no one else to speak on their behalf.

Mental Health Act 2007

This Act introduces amendments to the 1983 Mental Health Act; examples are given below.

• A single definition of mental disorder applies throughout the Act and abolishes references to 'categories of disorder'.

• A new 'appropriate medical treatment' test applies to all longer-term powers of detention. Patients now cannot be compulsorily detained or their detention continued unless medical treatment appropriate to their mental disorder is available (e.g. certain types of diagnosed personality disorder).

• A broader range of practitioners who can undertake the functions of the approved social worker and responsible medical officer (see Table 9.2).

• Community Treatment Orders (CTOs) allow psychiatrists to require patients to take supervised treatment in the community following discharge from hospital if they are seen as a risk to themselves or others. This is intended to prevent the 'revolving door' syndrome (i.e. patients leaving hospital and not continuing their treatment so that their health deteriorates and they need to be detained again).

• Patients can apply to displace their nearest relative and County Courts can displace a nearest relative if there are reasonable grounds for doing so. Nearest relative includes civil partner.

• Children and young people must be provided with mental health care in an environment suitable for their age and needs.

• Advocacy support is provided for anyone who is detained.

• Victims of violent and sexual crimes committed by mentally disordered offenders are to be told when offenders are discharged back into the community and have the right to make representations about their discharge.

The changing legal requirements for mental health work promise to alter clinical practice in this area.

Summary

• The definitions of mental disorder are particularly susceptible to social and cultural influences based on the theories of mind, normality and abnormality that people hold.

• The diagnosis of mental illness by health professionals is similarly influenced by cultural factors as evidenced by the diagnostic criteria used and the susceptibility to peer influence and labelling.

• Culture-bound syndromes are disorders specific to a particular group or locality.

• There are inequalities in the prevalence of psychiatric disorders. In the UK, women are more likely to suffer from depression, and men to commit suicide. Multifactorial circumstances explain the higher rates of mental disorder among some ethnic minority groups, for some of which institutional racism plays a part.

• Mental health policy has changed dramatically in the UK in the past 30 years, marked in particular by deinstitutionalization and the growth of community services. The Mental Health Act 1983 and its 2007 amendments, the National Service Framework 1999 and the Mental Capacity Act 2005 are examples of important contemporary social influences on psychiatric practice.

Further reading

Bhugra, D. and Bhui, K. (2001) African-Caribbeans and schizophrenia: contributing factors. *Advances in Psychiatric Treatment*, **7**: 283–91. http://apt.rcpsych.org/cgi/content/full/7/4/283.

Davies, T. and Craig, T. K. J. (eds) (1998) *ABC of Mental Health*. London: BMJ Books.

Department of Health (1999) *National Service Framework for Mental Health: Modern Standards and Service Models*. London: Department of Health._http://www.dh.gov.uk/en/Publicationsandstatistics/Publications/PublicationsPolicyAndGuidance/DH_4009598.

Harrison, P., Geddes, J. and Sharpe, M. (2005) *Lecture Notes: Psychiatry* (9th edn.). Oxford: Blackwell.

Helman, C. (2007) *Culture, Health and Illness* (5th edn.). London: Arnold, Chapter 10: Cross-cultural psychiatry.

Howard, P. and Bogle, J. (2005) *Lecture Notes: Medical Law and Ethics*. Oxford: Blackwell, Chapter 6: Mental health.

McKenzie, K. and Bhui, K. (2007) Institutional racism in mental health care. *British Medical Journal*, **334**: 649–50.

Nazroo, J. Y., Edwards, A. C. and Brown, G. W. (1998) Gender differences in the prevalence of depression: artefact, alternative disorders, biology or roles? *Sociology of Health and Illness*, **20(3)**: 312–30.

Rogers A. and Pilgrim, D. (2000) *A Sociology of Mental Health and Illness* (3rd edn.). Maidenhead: Open University Press.

Rosenhan, D. (1973) On being sane in insane places. *Science*, **179**: 250–8.

Singleton, N., Bumpstead, R., O'Brien, M., Lee, A. and Meltzer, H. (2001) *Psychiatric Morbidity among Adults Living in Private Households 2000*. London: The Stationery Office. http://www.statistics.gov.uk/downloads/theme_health/psychmorb.pdf.

Useful websites

http://www.mind.org.uk/index.htm MIND (National Association for Mental Health)

http://www.rcpsych.ac.uk/Royal College of Psychiatrists

http://www.mentalhealth.org.uk/Mental Health Foundation

Chapter 10

Disability and society

Introduction

One of the fundamental categorizations of people is into those who are 'able' and those who are 'disabled'. However, the nature of this division and how it is made varies widely across cultures and among peoples. For this reason, it is difficult to estimate how many people with disabilities there are in the UK, although disability of some sort is self-reported by 8.6 million people aged 16 and over, 15% of the population. Like chronic illness (see Chapter 12), the number of disabled people in the UK is likely to increase as the population ages, since the incidence of disability increases with age – 33% of 50–60 year olds report some form of disability. Disabled people form a higher proportion of those using health services. Many of the problems associated with disability are the result of prejudices and ignorance among the 'abled'. For example, the classic sign and symbol of disability is the wheelchair (Figure 10.1), although only about 8% of people classed as disabled in the UK use one.

Inequalities in the health of disabled people abound. Various barriers to disabled people accessing health care on an equal footing with people who are non-disabled have been identified, despite the efforts of legislation such as the Disability Discrimination Act 1995 to 'level the playing field'. People with disabilities are frequently subject to social exclusion in employment, transport and other forms of social interaction.

During the last 30 years, in response to the social exclusion they have experienced, a 'civil rights' movement among disabled people has done a lot to raise their profile and question the assumptions made by the non-disabled about them. Numerous self-help groups and organizations controlled and run by disabled people have been established worldwide, and are at the forefront of what has come to be known as the 'disabled movement'. Disabled activists, among others, question the way in which disabled people are often seen as people with 'needs' which for other people are 'rights'. For example, most people would regard access to a toilet as a right rather than a need, although making a toilet accessible for disabled people is often seen as a need rather than a right.

How disabled people see themselves and are seen by health care professionals has important implications for health care delivery. As with some chronic health conditions (see Chapter 12), the time that disabled people spend as a 'patient' is only a small fraction of their life as a whole, and

Lecture Notes: *The Social Basis of Medicine*, 1st edition. By Andrew Russell. Published 2009 by Blackwell Publishing. ISBN: 978-1-4051-3912-0

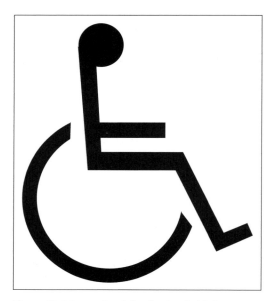

Figure 10.1 International sign for the disabled.

What is disability?

Medical model

The WHO, in its 1980 International Classification of Impairments, Disabilities and Handicaps (ICIDH) defined disability as 'any restriction or lack of ability to perform an activity in the manner or within the range considered normal for a human being'. Disability was seen as arising from impairment, defined as 'any loss or abnormality of psychological, physiological or anatomical structure or function'. Handicap, the WHO continued, was 'a disadvantage for a given individual, resulting from an impairment or disability, that limits or prevents the fulfilment of a role that is normal (depending on age, sex and social and cultural factors) for that individual'.

The ICIDH was widely criticized for identifying impairment as the determining factor in disability and the deprivations associated with it. Disability was presented as an entirely individual problem tied to the functional limitations of people with impairments: it was almost as if the victims were being 'blamed' for their problem. Rightly or wrongly, this has been called the 'medical model' of disability, although the validity of such a model is widely contested. Apart from the problem of defining what is 'normal' or 'abnormal' in each case, this model is silent about the environmental and/or social factors that are imposed on people with impairments and which can be much more 'disabling' than any limitations associated with the impairment itself. As such, the ICIDH provided a contested model, with definitions of disability and handicap that are now out of date.

in clinical contexts they may prefer to be regarded as a client, or a customer, rather than a patient. Furthermore, unlike people with chronic health conditions, most of the time disabled people do not see themselves as 'ill'. In this light, disabled people may see the health care they receive as oppressive, custodial and controlling, and this requires sensitivity from health and social care providers of all sorts.

The World Health Organization (WHO) and Disabled People's International are two examples of international organizations active in the field of defining and debating the terms used to describe and understand disability and in promoting the rights of people with disabilities. In the UK, the Disability Discrimination Act aims to improve the position of disabled people in society, and cultural values are also altering slowly. In the field of medicine, disability is not only an issue of 'able' doctors and some 'disabled' patients; in recent years disabled people have questioned the assumption that disability is incompatible with professional competence in medicine, and as a result the numbers of 'disabled' doctors is increasing.

Social model

The social model of disability starts from the premise that social discrimination and the barriers disabled people experience can have far more negative consequences for them than the impairment itself. In order to counteract the pernicious influence of the medical model of disability, the Union of the Physically Impaired against Segregation (UPIAS) defined disability as 'the disadvantage or restriction of activity caused by a contemporary social organization which takes little or no account of people who have physical impairments and thus excludes them from participation in the mainstream of social activities'. This definition acknowledges the reality of impairment, but focuses on the relationship of this impairment not to the individual but to society. In other words, disability is not seen as an individual problem as much as a social or civil rights issue similar to gender, race and sexuality – a problem caused by the fact that people with impairments are discriminated against, segregated and denied full, participative citizenship.

Note that the UPIAS (an organization founded in 1972 and disbanded in 1990) was only talking about the physically impaired, and their definition was subsequently extended by Disabled People's International to include intellectual impairments, sensory impairments and mental distress. For the Disabled Awareness in Action network, disability is simply 'the social consequences of having an impairment'.

In recent years, there has been some debate about whether the social model truly encompasses the reality and personal experience of impairment. Out of the medical model that (in physical terms) people are disabled by their bodies came its antithesis – the disabled rights movement's assertion that people are disabled by society, not by their bodies. There has been some recent convergence of these two opposing models in the view that people are disabled by society as well as by their bodies.

Functional model

In order to answer criticisms of its 'medical' model, in 2002 the WHO created a new International Classification of Functioning, Disability and Health (the ICF). This defines disability as the outcome of the interaction between a person with an impairment and the environmental and attitudinal barriers he or she may face. This definition attempts to shift the focus from disability as an individual problem towards disability as the outcome of impairment, activity limitation (function) and restrictions on participation. These three issues may be dealt with preventively or with an intervention (Table 10.1).

In this model, impairments lend themselves to medical interventions, activity limitation to rehabilitative interventions and participation restriction to social and environmental interventions.

Table 10.1 The WHO's International Classification of Functioning, Disability and Health (ICF).

	Intervention	Prevention
Impairment	Medical treatment/care	Prevention of the development of
	Medication	further activity limitations
	Surgery	
Activity limitation	Assistive devices	Preventive rehabilitation
	Personal assistance	Prevention of the development of
	Rehabilitation therapy	participation restrictions
Participation restriction	Accommodation	Environmental change
	Public education	Employment strategies
	Anti-discrimination legislation	Accessible services
	Universal design	Universal design
		Lobbying for change

The ICF thus reflects the idea that people are disabled by society and by their bodies, and is in some ways a compromise between the medical and social models.

Types of impairment

Given the disagreements over definition, a list of the different types of impairment is hard to produce, and such a list overlaps with chronic health conditions in some areas. A list compiled by the Department of Health includes among people with impairments those who have:

- Blindness or partial sight
- Deafness or are hard of hearing
- Heart conditions
- Epilepsy
- Continence problems
- Insulin-dependent diabetes
- Learning difficulty
- Down's syndrome
- Dyslexia
- Arthritis
- Mental health problems
- Need of a wheelchair
- Restricted growth

Case study: Ill health in people with learning difficulties

People with learning difficulties have higher rates of ill health and hence higher levels of morbidity and mortality. For example, it is estimated that people with learning difficulties are 58 times more likely to die before the age of 50 than the population as a whole. The burden of morbidity faced by people who find learning difficult is serious not only in its own right, but also because undiagnosed and untreated conditions are likely to have a disproportionately large impact when a person's functioning is already compromised, and to further inhibit that person's learning and potential for independent living.

Apart from specific physical illnesses associated with certain disabilities (e.g. cardiac valve disease in people with Down's syndrome), the prevalence of certain other conditions is higher in people with learning difficulties, for example:

- *Epilepsy* – increased incidence with severity of learning difficulty. May be due to same underlying cause as the learning difficulty. Can further compromise cognitive ability through seizure activity or side-effects of medication.
- *Sensory impairments* – adequate hearing and vision are important for psychomotor development, cognitive achievements and social/emotional development. Recognition and treatment of such impairments can significantly improve communication and learning ability. Excess earwax is particularly common and simple to treat.
- *Obesity* – may further increase stigma, as well as predispose to other health problems.
- *Gastrointestinal problems* – e.g. reflux oesophagitis, *Helicobacter pylori*, carcinoma, constipation.
- *Respiratory problems* – chest infections are particularly common.
- *Cerebral palsy* – especially in those with more severe learning difficulty.
- *Orthopaedic problems* – joint contractures, osteoporosis.
- *Dermatological problems.*
- *Psychiatric problems* (see Chapter 9).

Reasons why people with learning difficulties have higher rates of ill health
- Conditions that result from the same underlying cause as the person's learning difficulty (e.g. cerebral palsy due to hypoxic brain damage).
- Later presentation of illness.
- Poor access to screening – for example, only 3% of women with learning difficulties take up cervical screening compared with a general population uptake of 85%.
- Poor access to health services.
- Incomplete investigations of symptoms (assessment) and delay in treatment.
- Discrimination and prejudice in health care.

Points of view

- Short-sightedness (myopia) is an impairment not normally associated with disability. Why?
- Dyslexia – disability or difference?

The main factors in discrimination against disabled people

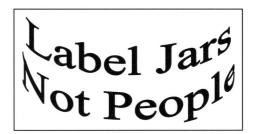

Figure 10.2 One of the slogans of People First.

Type of discrimination	Examples
Cultural	Language, e.g. invalid; handicapped; spastic; cripple; mongol; moron Images of the disabled
Social	Educational segregation
Economic	Unemployment; inadequate or no welfare benefits
Physical	Access in built environment – housing, transport
Behavioural	Abuse and violence, staring, lack of friendship and intimacy

Cultural discrimination

Language is by its very nature divisive. By naming someone as one thing, we are not naming them as another. Thus to call someone 'disabled' is to distinguish them from someone who is not disabled, usually in a negative way. This process, whereby descriptive words attached to people – such as the word 'disabled' itself – influences the attitudes and behaviours of others towards them, is known as labelling (see Chapter 2). People First, an organization run by and for people with learning difficulties, argues that people with such difficulties are disabled by society, and chooses to use the term 'learning difficulty' rather than 'learning disability' to communicate the idea that

learning support needs change over time (Figure 10.2).

Negative labelling may have the effect of increasing the characteristics associated with that label, either because of the tendency people have to live up to the expectations others have of them or because of the increased surveillance or segregation associated with the word, which increases the predicted behaviour (see Chapter 2). The very term 'disabled' may lead to increasing amounts of 'learned helplessness' in the person thus labelled. Labels are usually given by people in authority to those who are not.

Attitudes towards disabled people are influenced by images of them presented in the media and elsewhere. These form the 'cultural representations' of the disabled and are part of our socialization. Doctors are not immune to or removed from this process (see Chapter 1). Until quite recently literature often portrayed villains or other undesirables as having disabilities, whereas heroes and heroines were almost invariably beautiful and physically fit.

In an effort to turn a negative label into something positive to be proud of, deaf people have started writing about themselves as members of the Deaf community (with a capital 'D'). This is intended to symbolize their self-respect, strength and importance.

Three common images of the disabled

Image	Commentary	Examples
Tragic, but brave and plucky	Used a lot in charity advertising – makes us feel sorry for the individual represented and thankful we are not like them; sometimes may triumph over their tragedy.	Dickens' 'Tiny Tim' Heidi's friend Clara (a wheelchair user) overcoming her handicap in the novel by Johanna Spyri
Sinister villain	One book on writing for the Hollywood film industry suggested: 'if you want to make your villain more interesting, make them disabled'.	Captain Hook (in *Peter Pan*) Long John Silver (in *Treasure Island*) Abu Hamza, the radical Moslem cleric (an amputee) Richard III (allegedly a hunchback)
'Super crip'	Compensatory abilities enable them to overcome the disadvantage posed by their impairment and put them on a pedestal. A lesson to us all – there's always someone worse off than you, so why moan?	Helen Keller (deaf/blind) Douglas Bader (double amputee war hero) Ironside (paralysed TV detective) Stephen Hawking (Cambridge professor who has motor neurone disease) Jeremiah in the Old Testament The Who's 'Tommy'

All three types of images are stereotypes of what is usually a much more mundane reality, yet they have a hold on public imagination. They act as powerful levers against regarding disabled people as like anyone else rather than as people defined by their impairment.

Social discrimination

> ### Educational segregation – the debate over special needs schooling
>
> Prior to 1970, many young people with learning difficulties were regarded as uneducable and given no formal education. Since then, the term 'special educational needs' or 'children with special needs' has come to the fore. Disabled people have mixed feelings about the use of the word 'special' when what it means is separate and segregated.
>
> The debate about special schools mirrors the conflict between 'medical' and 'social' models of disability, with proponents of schools for children with special needs (including sometimes children in such schools) arguing that they can provide services for children which are tailored to their individual needs and wants. Opposing this view, the inclusive schools movement argues that rather than building separate institutions, it is 'normal' schools themselves that need to change to accommodate children with special needs. Integration also gives disabled and non-disabled pupils experience of and hopefully friendships with each other, so reducing the cultural barriers outlined above.
>
> The Warnock Report 1978 set the direction of policy in favour of inclusion 'wherever possible'. The 1981 Education Act gave a number of opt-outs from inclusion, such as parental wishes, the efficient use of resources and the effect on other children. A government Green Paper in 1997 aimed to get more children with special needs into mainstream schools, a position strengthened by the Special Needs and Disability Act 2001. The Alliance for Inclusive Education is currently campaigning for the closure of all special schools by 2020. In 1984 there were 1,548 special schools serving 118,500 pupils in England; by 2006 the number of special schools had fallen by nearly a quarter and they were serving nearly 30,000 fewer children than before.
>
> However in 2006 Baroness Warnock suggested that inclusion had been taken too far, driven by ideology rather than what was best for the individual child. Inclusion can fail when a child finds social integration difficult, although sometimes it may be because the mainstream school has not worked hard enough or lacked sufficient resources to make it work. Physical needs tend to be easier to meet than emotional or behavioural ones, which can often impact negatively on other children where the child with emotional or behavioural problems is disruptive in class. Fewer special schools and places result in less choice being available to parents and their children.

Economic discrimination

Disabled people are twice as likely to be unemployed as non-disabled people and almost three times more likely to want to work but not to have a job. A recent survey found that 15% of disabled young people said they had been turned down for a paid job for reasons related to their disability or other health problems. Approximately 40% of the disabled people of working age (2.7 million people) receive incapacity benefits because of a health condition or disability, at a cost of more than £19 billion per year. A similar proportion of disabled people are in work. However, 41% of disabled people of working age lack educational qualifications compared to 18% of the non-disabled and it has been calculated that incomes of households where at least one person is disabled are 20–30% lower than average. Yet the average cost of adjusting a workplace to make it more suitable for a disabled employee is small (only £184); the most commonly cited barrier to employment is supervisor knowledge of what adjustments need to be made.

Welfare benefits have historically always been very low to discourage 'scroungers' and people 'playing the system'. All disabled people are entitled to Disability Living Allowance (DLA), a benefit to help with their care costs and mobility needs. To be eligible for DLA-funded care, a person must require attention in connection with their bodily functions, or supervision to avoid a substantial danger. These can be in the day, at night, or both, and there is no lower age limit to claiming this part of the DLA. To be eligible for DLA Mobility, a person must be aged three or over and be unable, or virtually unable, to walk, or require guidance or supervision when walking outdoors. Receipt of DLA may entitle someone (or their carer) to claim Income Support, Housing Benefit, Council Tax Benefit, Working Families Tax Credit or Disabled Person's Tax Credit.

One of the most important policy developments for disabled people is the Community Care (Direct Payments) Act, which became law in 1997. This gave local authorities a mechanism to make cash payments direct to disabled people aged between 18 and 64 so that they could choose and pay for the social care services they wanted rather than having services imposed on them. An example is a disabled person employing someone as a personal assistant rather than as a carer. Direct payments challenge commonly held views that link disability and dependence. They have been slow to be implemented, however, particularly for those with learning difficulties and mental health problems. People have to consent to receiving direct payment, and giving such consent can be difficult for those with learning difficulties. Ethnic minorities have also been slow in taking up direct payments. Since 1997 the Act has been extended to enable direct payments to be an option for many more groups, including the carers of disabled children.

Physical discrimination

Paris, the disabling city?

The experience of being disabled is very different in different urban centres, in no small part due to the physical (built) environment and how much it enables disabled people to move about on a par with non-disabled people. The French capital has a poor track record with regard to accessibility for people with limited mobility. The following are among the problems experienced by mobility-impaired people visiting Paris.
- Wheelchair-intolerant, cobblestone streets.
- Metro stations either without lifts or with lifts that are frequently out of order.
- Café toilets in basements only accessible by a narrow spiral staircase.
- Hotels without lifts.

The experience of going to Paris for those with limited mobility can thus be something of an obstacle course and provides a graphic example of the social model of disability – it is the built environment that is disabling. Is London any better?

Behavioural discrimination

Disabled people are likely to experience a number of types of behavioural discrimination. They are twice as likely to be the victims of violent crime compared to non-disabled people. They often find themselves stared at. However, perhaps more profoundly troubling to disabled people is the loneliness and lack of intimacy that many experience and the assumption held by many non-disabled people, for whatever reason, that people with disabilities are asexual. In fact, there seems to be something of a taboo in society concerning discussions of disability and sex. Such an attitude is unsustainable given the social model of disability.

Case study: Treloar College's 'sexuality policy'

Treloar is a college in Hampshire for older teenagers with physical disabilities. In October 2007 the college announced a new sexuality policy, SAFE (Sexuality and Further Education). It was developed after a girl, severely disabled with cerebral palsy, asked a counsellor whether it was all right to fancy someone or whether society would find it disgusting.

The SAFE policy is a three-page document expressing the right of students to pursue physical and sexual relationships, assisted physically and emotionally by specially trained staff. Its focus is on dignity and respect, as well as providing information on safe sex. It marks a radical departure for the college, since in the past students were expelled if found engaging in sexual activity. For some young people with disabilities, even to hold hands, cuddle or kiss is impossible without help, and before the policy was introduced, many students rarely experienced touch other than with carers. It was as if sensuality was prohibited. Among the kinds of statements to which college staff can now respond sympathetically are:

'I know I am going to die in a couple of years and I would like a relationship before that.'

'I fancy someone of the same sex.'

'I have erections because I am a 17-year-old boy, but I have no hand control.'

The policy was two years in the making. Issues the college has had to deal with in developing it included the following:

- Some staff were so vehemently opposed to the idea that they refused to put up posters in their departments canvassing people's opinions. Even when the policy was finally agreed, one member of staff was so upset that she resigned.
- Legal advice was necessary concerning wording – for example, helping underage pupils with learning disabilities to have sex would be against the law.
- Establishing safeguards to make sure students were not 'coerced, exploited or manipulated' by their peers, and to set a clear boundary between 'assisting' pupils and becoming a participant.

The fundamental principle of the policy is that students over 18 are adults, and hence they should be enabled to do anything that a young adult who is not disabled would do, as long as it is legal and licensed, without passing moral judgements. In one case, for example, a student was permitted to visit a strip club before he died; another involved the purchase of erotic magazines and DVDs. It would be legal for a student to hire a prostitute, but if a member of staff made the phone call for him, that would be illegal as it would be classed as procurement.

Young people who, because of their disability, are likely to die in their twenties may express more intense sexual desires than people who are non-disabled. As one young person expressed it, 'We don't have much time left. We have to live our 77 years in 20.' One couple, both aged 20 and who used electric wheelchairs, were assisted in their relationship by a support worker, but they still found their love life frustrating. If they wanted to hug, they had to book time with their support worker, wait for her and a mattress to be brought in, and be assisted into position before they were left alone.

Other colleges for the disabled are likely to follow Treloar's lead, and the hospice movement is also interested. Meanwhile, the 17-year-old girl whose comment stimulated the development of the policy got a boyfriend, and subsequently became engaged and got married.

Recent legislation in support of disabled people

The Disability Discrimination Act 1995

The Disability Discrimination Act (DDA) introduced a number of measures that attempt to overcome those forms of discrimination against the disabled that are amenable to legal manipulation. It is based on a fairly medical definition of disability – a physical or mental impairment that has a substantial and long-term adverse effect on a person's ability to carry out normal day-to-day activities.

The DDA is designed to protect disabled people in the areas of:

- Employment.
- Access to goods, facilities and services.
- The management, buying or renting of land or property.
- Education.
- Transport, allowing the government to set minimum standards to assist disabled people in using public transport easily.

The Act has been amended since its introduction. For service providers (i.e. businesses and organizations, including the NHS):

- Since December 1996 it has been *unlawful to treat disabled people less favourably* than other people for a reason related to their disability.
- Since October 1999 they have had to make *reasonable adjustments* for disabled people, such as providing extra help or making changes to the way they provide their services.
- From 2004 they have had to make reasonable adjustments to the *physical features* of their premises to overcome physical barriers to access.
- From December 2006 all public bodies have had a duty to promote disability equality via a local Disability Equality Scheme and action plan which disabled people must have been involved in producing.

For education providers new duties came into effect in September 2002 under Part IV of the DDA as amended by the Special Educational Needs and Disability Act 2001 (SENDA). These require schools, colleges, universities, providers of adult education and youth services to ensure that they do not discriminate against disabled people. The duty for education providers to make auxiliary aids available, by way of reasonable adjustment, came into force in September 2003.

Making 'reasonable adjustments' means doing things to anticipate the needs of disabled people rather than simply reacting as needs arise. Account is taken of the size of the organization and the cost and practicality of the measures.

The Community Care (Direct Payments) Act 1996

The Community Care (Direct Payments) Act 1996 came into force in April 1997. It gave councils the power (not duty) to provide Direct Payments (cash) to individuals assessed as needing community care services. Supported by the National Centres for Independent Living (NCIL), part of a worldwide network of disabled people dissatisfied with professional services, disabled people had run a campaign for the right to live independently in the community. Independence for NCIL was not about being able to do activities unaided, but about choice over where and how to live, who provides assistance, and control over when, where and how that assistance was provided. Local authorities were expected to work in partnership with disabled people, giving them as much choice as possible while at the same time ensuring that the individual's needs were being met and that public money was being used appropriately and cost-effectively. The Carers and Disabled Children's Act 2000 extended Direct Payments to carers over the age of 16 years providing a substantial amount of care to an adult, people with parental responsibility for a disabled child who provide a substantial amount of care on a regular basis to that child, and disabled young people aged 16 and 17 years. In 2003, the Health and Social Care Act altered the status of the 1996 legislation, making Direct Payments a duty of councils.

Direct Payments have proved very popular, although some people express frustration that they cannot be used to buy health service provision such as physiotherapy. This may change in the future.

Disability and the culture of medicine

Health professionals are not immune to the often discriminatory attitudes of society towards disability and their roots in prejudice or simply lack of insight into the lives of disabled people. Disabled people in turn may come to resent their treatment at the hands of health professionals, with some seeing providers as parasites using the tools of their trade to assess clients, define their problems and needs, and evaluate the efficacy of solutions in a self-perpetuating fashion. There are also themes specific to the culture of medicine which, because they are at odds with the perceptions of many disabled people, can detrimentally affect the way in which the disabled and their carers are treated, as well as their attitudes to the medical profession.

Three cultural themes in medicine that can be problematic when dealing with the disabled:

1 Emphasis on curing disease.

2 Suggestion that what cannot be cured should be prevented.

3 Linking health problems to impairment (diagnostic overshadowing).

Emphasis on curing disease

The emphasis on curing disease presents issues similar to those that arise with the care of the chronically ill (see Chapter 12), because disabled people cannot normally be 'cured'. Sometimes quite risky procedures may be carried out as if they are some kind of indispensable medical surgery when in fact their goal is simply to normalize a less than perfect body. Examples of interventions whose value is questioned, the value of which are questioned by many disabled people, include cochlear implants, lengthening limbs, straightening body parts and plastic surgery for people with Down's syndrome.

Should what cannot be cured be prevented?

Case study: Screening for Down syndrome

Down's syndrome (trisomy 21) is the most common chromosomal abnormality, occurring in approximately 1 in 700 births. There are approximately 60,000 people with Down syndrome living in the UK. Since it is a genetic condition, it cannot be cured and the question arises as to whether it can or should be prevented.

A number of conditions are associated with Down syndrome:
- Chest and sinus infections in babies
- Some degree of learning disability, with milestones reached later than other children of their age
- Heart problems (in up to 50% of cases), ranging from minor heart murmurs to more serious abnormalities, which may require surgery
- Mild to moderate hearing loss
- Visual problems such as squints and long- or short-sightedness
- Increased chance of developing Alzheimer's disease in later life.

The average life expectancy of a person with Down syndrome is approximately 50 years.

Screening tests (either blood or ultrasound) are available for mothers who are at increased risk of having a baby with Down's syndrome (usually older women) and are usually done at 15–22 weeks of pregnancy. If these tests indicate a higher risk pregnancy, the results can be verified with diagnostic tests called chorionic villus sampling (CVS) and amniocentesis. These give a definitive answer as to whether or not a foetus has Down syndrome, but amniocentesis carries a 1% chance of miscarriage and CVS a 1–2% chance.

Various criticisms have been made of screening services by parents and people with Down syndrome themselves. Issues raised include:
- If parents have no intention of terminating the pregnancy if a diagnosis is made, there is little point in being screened.
- Promoting screening for Down syndrome gives people with the condition a message that it would have been better if they had not been born, a painful and threatening idea with which most would disagree. Others argue that the prevention of impairment through screening and the rights of the disabled are not incompatible.

Diagnostic overshadowing

The disability faced by an individual can sometimes become a mask for more serious problems. A doctor who is preoccupied with the disability may ignore the actual symptoms that a patient presents with. This is known as diagnostic overshadowing. For example, a patient who is wheelchair-bound and overweight may suffer from aches and pains that the doctor attributes to the weight problem when in fact they may indicate a spreading melanoma. A patient with disabling mental health problems who complains of physical health problems may also find their difficulties overlooked. Diagnostic overshadowing has been particularly noticeable in studies of people with learning disabilities where there are communication difficulties. Therefore when a person with learning disabilities presents with a new behaviour, or existing ones escalate, it is important to consider:

- *Physical problems* – pain or discomfort, e.g. from ear infection, toothache, constipation, reflux oesophagitis, deterioration in vision or hearing.
- *Psychiatric causes* – depression, anxiety, psychosis, dementia.
- *Social causes* – change in carers, bereavement, abuse.

Case study: Diagnostic overshadowing in the obese

'When I went to the doctor with chronic pain in my shoulder, rosacea, eczema and bouts of nausea and vomiting – clear symptoms of a diseased gall bladder – my GP simply Googled the nearest Weight Watchers class and gave me the time and date of the next meeting.'

Madeleine White, *Guardian Weekend*,
1 March 2008

Ways of better serving people with disabilities

There are numerous ways in which a clinician can improve the service they provide for people with disabilities. Many of the suggestions that follow may seem like common sense, but it is surprising how often they are overlooked, thus perpetuating the attitudes and barriers of the wider world within clinical settings. Doctors need to provide a model of leadership that offers a high quality of service with respect and dignity for all patients, including those who are disabled. Staff training in disability equality and awareness enables better communication with and understanding of the needs of disabled people. This is particularly true for those who have first contact with patients (e.g. receptionists, switchboard operators, practice nurses and therapists). Disabled people are often the best placed to deliver this training.

Broadening the benefits

It should be noted that the provision of facilities that are mindful of the needs of disabled people will also be of benefit to a far wider patient group. For example:
- Everyone benefits from clear signage.
- Access ramps to a surgery will be helpful to those with pushchairs as well as to wheelchair users.
- Easy to read materials will be of use to those whose first language is not English as well as to those with reading difficulties.

Publicity materials and documentation

- Use a large font size in publicity materials and provide other formats, such as Braille or audio cassettes, on request, making it clear on the printed documents that alternative formats are available.
- Use clear English in documents and on websites, with pictures or symbols like Widgit, Makaton or Signalong.
- Describe the facilities to help disabled people, such as details about physical access and the arrangements you can make for people requiring British Sign Language (BSL) interpreters or lip speakers. Highlight in publicity materials that you want to assist disabled service users to access services, and that you are happy to discuss any additional requirements they may have.
- Provide a fax number, email address and Textphone number on all publicity materials and

documentation so that people who have difficulties using the telephone can make an appointment, and make sure staff know how to use these alternatives.

Making an appointment

- Find out the service requirements a disabled person has at the time of making an appointment and pass these on to the appropriate people for action.
- Enable patients to discuss their requirements confidentially and discreetly.
- Note such requirements in the patient's records (with their consent).
- Set a longer appointment time to allow for any possible barriers a disabled service user might face, particularly if they are using the service for the first time.

Examples of particular service requirements patients might have

- An adult patient with a learning disability may wish for a consultation without their family or support worker present (although in other contexts their knowledge and support can be invaluable).
- A deaf person may wish a particular 'signer' to be used.
- An adjustable bed may be needed for a disabled patient who has difficulty and needs assistance getting onto and off an examination or treatment couch.
- Patients with learning disabilities may need to meet several times in order for rapport and trust to be established.

From home to clinic

- For people whose disability makes it difficult for them to attend the surgery or clinic, a home visit may be preferable.
- Help with travel arrangements may be appropriate, and information about local transport and details about disabled access will be useful.
- Make available a number of clearly marked, accessible car parking bays close to the entrance of your premises, and monitor them so that they are only used by people with disabilities. If there is no accessible parking, provide a drop-off nearby which allows level access to the entrance.
- The entrance should be easy to find from the street, car park or other routes to the building. Access routes and signs should be free of obstacles

and easily visible after dark. The entrance should be well lit, with level access or a ramp and handrails.
- Easy opening, preferably automatic, doors are better for everyone, and these should have clear, contrasting safety markings.
- If there is a call bell or entry phone, this should be at a height accessible to wheelchair users. If an intercom system is used, a member of staff should be available to help disabled users.

At reception

- Make sure reception desks are clearly visible and at heights that are suitable for disabled people who might be standing or seated.
- Consider installing auxiliary aids such as an induction loop system for hearing aid users.
- Glass screens at the reception counter can reflect the light and cause difficulties for visually impaired people as well as making an additional barrier for someone who is deaf or hard of hearing.
- Use a flexible approach.

Examples of a flexible approach at reception

- If desk height options are limited, staff should come out from behind the desk or hatch to assist a wheelchair user or someone of restricted height.
- A patient may need to be escorted from the reception to the treatment area if they are visually impaired.

Internal arrangements

- Good lighting and colour contrast in internal decoration help all service users.
- Make sure internal signage is clear, well lit with Braille or pictograms, and is positioned to be visible to both disabled and non-disabled.
- Waiting areas should create a calm, welcoming environment.
- Chairs should be of various sizes, some with high backs and/or arm rests, and of a different colour from the walls and carpets to provide a contrast (as an aid to the visually impaired).
- Rearrange some seating to make space for wheelchairs, prams or children's play areas, and have sufficient space for a wheelchair user to be alongside a seated companion.

• Make announcement systems both visible and audible for people with hearing or visual impairments; staff can usually alert a patient of their appointment turn by approaching them discreetly to inform them of it.

• An accessible toilet can double up as an infant changing facility or other personal care facility.

• Use light colour schemes in bathrooms with some contrast at floor or wall level to help prevent a visually impaired person from tripping over or catching themselves on rails and fittings.

• Fire alarm systems need to alert everyone, including people with hearing impairments.

• Training in emergency evacuation procedures should include how to deal with service users who need extra help.

• Specific aids for disabled people, such as 'evac-chairs', should be located on accessible upper floors and staff should be trained in their use.

In the consultation

Possible reasons why a disabled person may have problems communicating:

• Intellectual impairment leading to problems comprehending and processing information.

• Sensory difficulties (hearing, vision).

• Problems in understanding social interaction (e.g. autism).

• Speech problems (e.g. with articulation).

• Prior experience of others not listening to or valuing what they are trying to communicate.

Ways in which the doctor can assist in communicating with disabled patients

• Allow someone with a disability extra time to describe their symptoms.

• Maintain patience and value what is being communicated.

• Be sensitive to possible non-verbal cues and alternative communication strategies if verbal communication is difficult (e.g. use of symbols, sign language).

• Communicate directly with the patient unless informed otherwise, even when a disabled patient has a family member or support worker with them.

• Explain things clearly in an appropriate way using plain, simple English where possible. In the case of patients with learning disabilities, books are available that use pictures to explain common health problems and procedures (e.g. breast screening).

• If a deaf patient is accompanied by a sign language interpreter, pause frequently while you are explaining a diagnosis to allow enough time for the interpreter to finish signing.

• Take time to explain your diagnosis and treatment to disabled patients – in particular, allow extra time to give instructions for taking medication.

• Consider capacity and consent issues carefully (see Chapter 9).

Follow-up

• Offer annual health checks, with screening, for disabled people at high risk, such as those with long-term mental health problems or learning disabilities (sometimes community learning disability teams may do this).

• Provide information about which local pharmacies offer a pick-up and deliver service to disabled people. Alternatively, telephone orders of repeat prescriptions and posting them to the service user may be appropriate.

• Get regular feedback from all patients including disabled people, through feedback forms including specific questions about how service requirements were recognised and addressed. Make arrangements to help people who have difficulty reading or writing to fill in the form.

Disabled people as health professionals

Disability does not simply concern patients. Disability legislation applies to the health professions as well and raises interesting questions concerning competency and what it means to be a doctor.

> **Case study: Heidi Cox**
>
> In 1992, Heidi Cox had to leave St George's Hospital Medical School after an accident left her disabled. She subsequently decided to resume her training and enrolled on a course specially adapted to her needs at Oxford University. However, the General Medical Council (GMC) decided that it could not approve a specially adapted course that would result in the achievement of a lesser degree of skill and knowledge. With the backing of the Disability Rights Commission, Cox took the GMC to a discrimination employment tribunal on the grounds that it was discriminating against disabled people according to the 1995 Disability Discrimination Act (DDA).
>
> The GMC's concern was not with the health or disability of a medical student but with her ability to achieve all the outcomes listed in 'Tomorrow's Doctors', which were a prerequisite for registration. Cox, the GMC argued, would not be able to do cardiopulmonary resuscitation (CPR) and hence would not have achieved all the outcomes required. Patient safety is a duty, and there is no question that there are limits to who can be a doctor and what speciality they can practise. But from a tradition that medical students must succeed at everything, it is now accepted that physical disabilities may prevent a doctor doing certain tasks, but not others. For example, a serious visual impairment precludes surgery but not the entire medical spectrum. Traditionally, for example, every doctor has been expected to be able to perform CPR, although once registered their competency in it was never reassessed.
>
> The case of Heidi Cox has led to a change in procedures whereby it is accepted that where a person's disability might prevent it, a modified form of CPR can be used, or special arrangements made to ensure the person concerned is not left alone without a colleague who could perform CPR.

The Special Educational Needs and Disability Act 2001

This Act gave disabled students the right not to be discriminated against in education or training. With this legislation, the GMC had to review the required competencies for medicine to make sure they were not discriminatory. Universities were required to make reasonable adjustments to enable the achievement of the competencies by disabled students. Assessment methods in particular were highlighted to ensure that disabled students were not being excluded simply on the basis of a type of test.

Summary

- Disabled people are more likely to have morbidity problems than the general population, and their numbers are likely to increase in the future.
- Disability stems from impairment; however, there is a fundamental difference between 'medical' models that see disability as a problem of individual incapacity and 'social' models that see incapacity in society's response to disability. Functional models of disability attempt to reconcile these opposing viewpoints.
- There are various types of discrimination against disabled people – cultural, social, economic, behavioural and practical.

- Recent legislation has sought to improve the rights of the disabled and their access to facilities.
- Medicine is not dissociated from the types of discrimination against disabled people found in wider society, and some disabled patients may feel or express resentment against the profession.
- At all stages of the patient's journey from home to the clinic and back again, there are ways in which services can be made more 'disability-friendly'. This is part of a patient-centred approach to care.
- It has become marginally easier for people with disabilities to become doctors, through some recent legislative test cases.

Further reading

Alderson, P. (2001) Down's syndrome: cost, quality and value of life. *Social Science and Medicine*, **55**(5): 627–38.

Finkelstein, V. (2004) The commonality of disability. In J. Swain et al. (eds) *Disabling Barriers – Enabling Environments* (2nd edn.). London: Sage.

French, S. (1993) Disability, impairment, or something in between. In J. Swain et al. (eds) *Disabling Barriers – Enabling Environments*. London: Sage.

Gosling, J. (2003) *Helping the Handicapped* (a web-based artwork series created for 'Sinnlos', Graz, Austria). http://www.sinnlos.st/help/eng/help1.htm.

Oliver, M. (1990) *The Politics of Disablement*. London: Macmillan.

Shakespeare, T. (2006) *Disability Rights and Wrongs*. London: Routledge.

Swain, J., French, S. and Cameron, C. (2003) *Controversial Issues in a Disabling Society*. Buckingham: Open University Press.

WHO (2002) *Towards a Common Language for Functioning, Disability and Health*. http://www3.who.int/icf/beginners/bg.pdf.

Useful resources

The Disabled Awareness in Action (DAA) network – 'an international human rights network, run for and by disabled people'. http://www.daa.org.uk/

The National Centre for Independent Living. http://www.ncil.org.uk/

People First. http://www.peoplefirstltd.com/index.php

Disability Rights Commission. Absorbed into the Equality and Human Rights Commission, October 2007. http://www.equalityhumanrights.com/en/Pages/default.aspx

'Books Beyond Words' series, Gaskell Books.

Chapter 11

Promoting health

Introduction

One of the reasons the 'medical model' of health or health as the absence of disease (see Chapter 2) is so called is that medicine is conventionally viewed as treating disease rather than promoting health. In terms of status, funding and personnel, far more is invested in therapeutic medicine than in preventive medicine. Yet in terms of benefit to society per pound spent, preventive medicine can achieve a lot more than therapeutic medicine in terms of saving lives and increasing overall health and well-being. Some doctors know little about the potential for preventing disease in their work and have an exaggerated view of the benefits of treatment, although such a view is becoming rarer. More and more emphasis is being put in policy circles on health promotion in clinical contexts (proactive medicine) over and above the imperative to 'treat the sick' (reactive medicine). Doctors need to take health promotion work seriously and see it as an integral part of what they do.

Lecture Notes: The Social Basis of Medicine, 1st edition. By Andrew Russell. Published 2009 by Blackwell Publishing. ISBN: 978-1-4051-3912-0

What is health promotion?
Methods of health promotion
Other ways of categorising health promotion

What is health promotion?

Health promotion has been defined as 'the process of enabling people to increase control over, and to improve, their health'. For the medical model of health, health promotion is about reducing the levels of disease and injury in society. The functional model of health suggests that health promotion involves improving people's ability to fulfil their social roles, while the idealist view of health sees it as increasing people's levels of physical, mental and social well-being (see Chapter 2). The medical model, in taking a 'negative' view of health, sees its achievement through avoiding the causes of disease (pathogens). The idealist model, with its 'positive' view of health, looks to embrace the causes of health (salutogens). Opinions differ as to what the nature of these salutogens may be. However, the Ottawa Conference on Health Promotion in 1986 (from which the definition of health promotion given above derives) identified a number of prerequisites for health which are necessary irrespective of what definition of health one subscribes to.

Prerequisites for health (from the Ottawa Conference 1986)

- Peace
- Shelter
- Education
- Food
- Income
- Stable ecosystem
- Sustainable resources
- Social justice
- Equity

Lack of one or more of these prerequisites, while not necessarily crucial in itself, is likely to deleteriously affect the health profile of an individual or a population.

Methods of health promotion

Disease prevention
Health protection
Health education

Disease prevention

Disease prevention is sometimes known as the 'medical' perspective on prevention because it can often take place or be arranged in clinical settings, particularly primary health care. Immunizations and screening services form a large part of the

medical work of disease prevention. Different levels can be identified (Table 11.1).

Disease prevention is based on an epidemiological understanding of causal mechanisms and hence has a relatively high status within the medical profession. Primary and secondary prevention are acknowledged as being cheaper than tertiary prevention. There have been some spectacular successes with disease prevention at the international level, such as the worldwide eradication of smallpox and near-eradication of polio. What is offered tends to be the result of top-down policy and planning by 'experts'. Sometimes where there is disagreement among 'experts', this can backfire, such as the public revolt in the UK against the MMR (measles, mumps and rubella) vaccine (see below). Another problem with disease prevention is that it is often aimed 'at' people rather than working 'with' them in a more empowering way. This can often involve implied (or overt) 'victim blaming' and negative attitudes, such as when smokers, pregnant teenagers or the obese are targeted.

Health protection

Health protection aims to protect individuals, groups and populations not only from infectious diseases, but also from environmental hazards such as chemical contamination or radiation.

Table 11.1 Levels of disease prevention.

Level	Aims	Requirements	Examples
Primary prevention	To prevent the onset of disease or injury and the development of risk factor(s)	Knowledge of causal mechanisms and natural history of disease	Use of hand-washing, antiseptics, barrier nursing, immunization, chemoprophylaxis (e.g. for malaria), vitamin supplements, health education to discourage uptake of smoking
Secondary prevention	To halt progress of disease in early (pre-clinical) stages	Methods to detect disease, diagnosis and effective treatment (e.g. screening)	Antenatal/child health care Screening for cervical cancer
Tertiary prevention	To treat or rehabilitate people with established disease or risk factor(s)	Methods to treat and rehabilitate, achieving demonstrable increase in quality of life	Physiotherapy; community support for housebound chronically ill; smoking cessation services

Case study: The Clean Air Act 1956

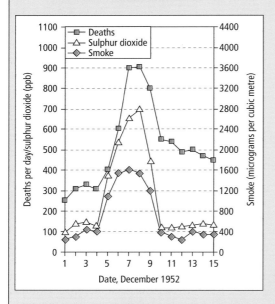

Figure 11.1 Mortality statistics during the great London smog of 1952.

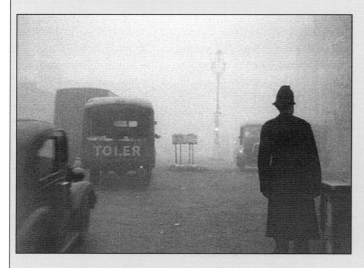

Figure 11.2 The London smog of December 1952.

In London in December 1952, a temperature inversion (where warmer air is above colder air closer to the ground, so preventing convection currents from rising) led to hundreds of tons of coal soot particulates and sulphur dioxide failing to rise and disperse, creating a yellow-grey 'pea soup' smog. This lasted five days before the weather changed and winds blew the smog away. During this period at least 4000 people died, with mortality from pneumonia and bronchitis increasing sevenfold.

As a result of this tragedy the government introduced the Clean Air Act authorizing local councils to set up smokeless zones and make grants to householders to convert their domestic heating from coal fires to heaters fuelled by gas, oil, smokeless fuel or electricity.

However, while the Act has had an undeniable positive effect on human health in the capital, in December 1991 another smog, this one caused by motor vehicle traffic, developed. It is estimated that 160 lives were claimed as a result; statistics on non-fatal illnesses were not kept.

Many public health-trained doctors work for the Health Protection Agency, set up in 2002 to provide an integrated approach to protecting the health of the public. Local Health Protection Units provide advice and support on a variety of issues.

Examples of health protection

- Communicable disease control
- Environmental hazard control (e.g. radiological, chemical and environmental)
- Major incident and emergency planning
- Promoting technologies that protect health, e.g.
  - Biotechnologies (e.g. genetic modification of food crops to enhance nutritional content)
  - Chemical technologies (e.g. fly sprays; antiseptic lotion)
  - Mechanical technologies (e.g. sewage disposal plants; electric cars; domestic water systems; smoke detectors)
  - Electronic technologies (e.g. flight control radar)
- Healthy public policy

Examples of mechanical technologies that improve road safety

- Pedestrian barriers
- School crossing patrols (and their 'lollipop sticks')
- Speed bumps and other traffic calming measures
- Speed cameras
- Speed limit signs
- Traffic islands
- Zebra and pelican crossings

Healthy public policy covers the local, regional, national and international policy-making that directly or indirectly acts to protect health. Examples include legal controls such as seat belt legislation to reduce road accident injury and deaths, fiscal controls such as raising taxation on alcohol as a means of reducing consumption, and other regulations and policies such as health and safety at work regulations.

Why legislate?

There have been recent debates around whether legislation is preferable to voluntary codes of practice concerning things such as the regulation of breast milk substitutes in developing countries or the provision of smoke-free areas in pubs. Opinion among public health researchers has generally shifted away from voluntary codes of practice, since they are often ineffective.

Advantages of legislation over voluntary codes of practice

- Uniquely comprehensive in coverage rather than based on piecemeal local agreements.
- Permanent (unless repealed or amended).
- Strong coercive power (e.g. through fines, imprisonment, public censure).
- Supported by plentiful resources to uphold the law (e.g. the police, environmental protection officers).
- Symbolic value (imparts a message about social priorities and moral standpoints).

Case study: The Health Improvement and Protection Act 2006

In 2005 the government introduced a parliamentary bill which included proposals for a ban on smoking in enclosed public places and workplaces in England. Such a proposal was the result of many years of lobbying by health
(continued on p. 152)

(continued)

organizations and pressure groups. Evidence for the harmful health effects of second-hand smoke inhalation became overwhelming, and countries such as Australia, Ireland and Scotland, as well as some US states (e.g. California) were successful in implementing smoke-free workplaces legislation. Several options were offered in the English bill: a comprehensive ban, a ban with exemptions or devolving the decision about whether or not to go 'smoke-free' to local authority level. The government initially favoured the ban with exemptions option, which proposed permitting private members' clubs and licensed premises that did not prepare or serve food ('wet pubs') to circumvent the legislation. However, by concentrating on the inequalities that would arise because of the geographical distribution of 'wet' pubs (which are found in predominantly working-class neighbourhoods) and how illogical it was, in health terms, to allow some workplaces to get round the legislation, lobbying was successful in convincing a majority of MPs to vote for the comprehensive ban. England went 'smoke-free' on 1 July 2007.

Smoking remains the principal cause of preventable death and ill health in the country, and so this is probably the single most important piece of health legislation for a generation.

Health education

Health education in the narrow sense enables people to increase their knowledge of, and hence it is assumed their control over, the determinants of health and health behaviours. In the broader sense health education is all the influences that determine knowledge, beliefs and behaviours concerning health, including its maintenance and restoration. These influences come from both formal and informal education in the family, school, the media and society at large, as well as in the special context of health service activities.

> **Health education**
> - Can be aimed at individuals or at whole populations.
> - Can be aimed at the general public or health professionals.
> - Can be simple or complex.
> - Has a rich theoretical background.
> - Is starting to become evidence-based.

Health professionals, including doctors, have an important role to play in the field of health education. Three main approaches can be identified (Table 11.2).

Table 11.2 Approaches to health education.

Approach	Aims	Characteristics	Examples
Propaganda	To change behaviour	May be untrue/use fear tactics Paternalistic, disempowering, short-termist	'AIDS: Don't Die of Ignorance' campaign launched in 1987
Information	To enable informed choice	Assumes knowledge leads to behaviour change Assumes information is needed Must be context-specific Often paternalistic	'Five a Day' nutrition leaflets
Empowerment	To facilitate development, confidence, self-esteem, autonomy and skills	Based on needs as defined by individuals and communities	'Reclaim the Night' poster advertising an event aimed at stopping violence against women

Resistance to health education

Irrational or differently rational? Why people may resist making health behaviour changes

In-depth interviews of 180 randomly sampled people in South Wales in the late 1980s found a well-established 'lay epidemiology' concerning the causes of heart disease. Along with public health messages concerning how to prevent coronary heart disease, people often had personal experience of those who had ignored such messages and 'lived to tell the tale'. Conversely, some could give examples of people with extremely healthy lifestyles who had died of a heart attack while still relatively young. Even though such deaths are relatively rare, they may loom large in public consciousness because they are dramatic, unexpected and premature. Such examples of luck, fate and destiny complicate people's views of the risks of heart disease and make health education problematic. Statistical evidence (e.g. that people who have a high-fat diet and/or smoke are more likely to die of heart disease than those who don't) flies in the face of individual cases that, for whatever reason, tend to figure highly in people's decision-making regarding health behaviour change.

Methods of health education

- Teaching, advising/counselling, advocacy.
- Adverts and programmes on TV/radio.
- Adverts and articles in newspapers/magazines.
- Leaflets and booklets; posters and billboards; stickers, badges, postmarks, stamps, labels.
- Any other novel ideas (see Figures 11.3 and 11.4).

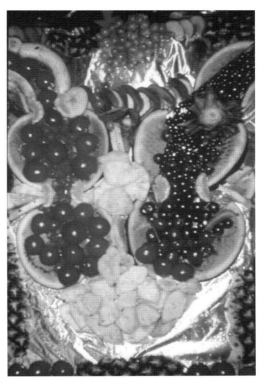

Figure 11.3 Fruit sculpture of the heart showing the four chambers with oxygenated and deoxygenated blood made in a public workshop led by Pioneer Projects Ltd. Photo: Alison Jones.

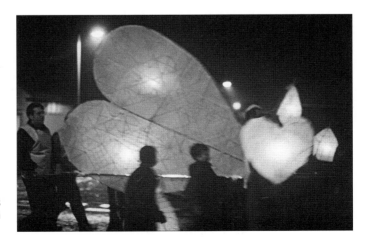

Figure 11.4 'Happy Hearts' lanterns event, a schools-based arts in health initiative (Source: Sharon Bailey).

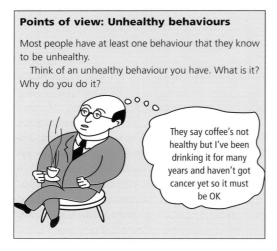
The relative 'need' to change – another reason why people may resist making health behaviour changes

The 'need' to make a specific change is based on what other needs a person may have. Sometimes the needs an individual perceives themselves as having may be different from those of a health professional. They may also be tempered by the different needs of those they live with. The felt needs of an individual (what they want) may be different from their expressed needs (what they demand). A hierarchy of needs has been identified which are sequential – the satisfaction of lower-order needs being a prerequisite for the satisfaction of higher-order ones (Figure 11.5).

Physiological needs: Food, water, warmth, sleep, air, sexuality.

Safety needs: Physical safety, economic security, freedom from threats, comfort, peace, familiarity, regularity and a secure home.

Love and belonging: Acceptance, group membership, affection from at least one other person.

Esteem: Feeling worthwhile and capable, recognition of talents, society values our contribution.

Self-actualization: Opportunities for innovation and creativity, ability to experience joy, development and use of potential.

Case study: Health promotion among the homeless

Homeless people are a heterogeneous group with a wide range of needs. The health status of the homeless is extremely poor compared to that of the general population. They are more likely to present at the third level of disease prevention rather than at the primary (prevention) or secondary (screening) levels. They are less likely to be registered with a primary health care facility and more likely to use an Accident and Emergency Department for their health care needs. As a result, they are often missed by approaches to health promotion that work through primary care.

The homeless are a good example of a group in which lower-level needs for things such as food, drink, warmth and shelter may compromise concern for higher-level needs such as the possibility of preventing illness in the future. As one commentator put it, 'one useful intervention might simply be to tell a homeless person where the nearest shelter or soup kitchen is'. Practical assistance, such as providing toothbrushes, sunhats, sunscreen lotion, clean socks and washing facilities, should supplement information about dental health, how to avoid sunstroke and hypothermia, caring for feet and general hygiene. The multiple needs of homeless people make collaborative working across sectors (e.g. primary care groups, housing services, voluntary agencies) the most effective way to deliver coordinated health promotion.

Stages of change model

The stages of change model is based on the observation that not everyone is ready to effect change in their behaviour at the same time, but that different stages of readiness can be identified. So prevalent is this pattern that the model is also known as the 'transtheoretical model' because it

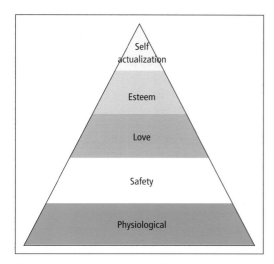

Figure 11.5 Maslow's hierarchy of needs.

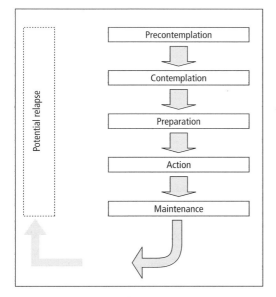

Figure 11.6 The stages of change model (Prochaska and Comente)

is applicable to all fields of human endeavour, not just health. Understanding the different stages is useful in identifying individuals who are ready to make a change and supporting them in that process in the most appropriate way.

Don't give up giving up.

Figure 11.7 Health promotion message for relapsing smokers.

Pre-contemplation: people at this stage are not seriously considering changing; they may have considered it and rejected the possibility, never have thought about it, or be thinking vaguely about making a change at some point in the future. If a health professional is involved at this point their goal is to get the person to consider changing their behaviour, preferably through discussing both the benefits and barriers faced in a personalized way.
Contemplation: when people are aware a problem exists and are seriously considering changing to a healthier behaviour. The role of the health professional is to encourage this process and make more concrete plans to achieve change.
Preparation: the individual is ready to try to change in the near future and is making preparations to do so. Such a person may find support useful, particularly in setting concrete plans, such as deciding when and where to make the change.
Action: the person 'takes the plunge' and attempts to change their behaviour consistently over a period of months. A clear goal, a realistic plan and rewards are useful, and the health professional can be particularly helpful when unexpected obstacles arise.
Maintenance: people work to maintain their behaviour change. Intervention from the health professional is usually minimal.
Relapse: where this occurs, the health professional provides support and encouragement to bring the person back to the preparation stage.

'Brief intervention' advice in primary care

'Brief interventions' are short (5–10 minutes) advice periods given by health professionals (such as GPs) with a view to promoting a healthy lifestyle or a lifestyle change. Evidence suggests that such interventions have a small but significant effect on some aspects of health behaviour (e.g.

quitting smoking and reducing alcohol consumption) but not others (e.g. taking more exercise).

Brief interventions for smokers

A quarter of the UK population smoke but giving up is hard: 70% of all smokers would like to give up, but only 3–4% will succeed using willpower alone. However, smoking cessation services offer a quit rate of up to 15%. The average number of attempts a smoker makes to give up smoking before succeeding is 3–4 (see Figure 11.7). Brief

advice from GPs to all smokers to quit has a small but significant effect on smoking cessation rates. Studies have shown that 40% of smokers make an attempt to quit after receiving advice from their GP, and 1–3 out of every 100 people receiving such information go on to give up smoking for at least six months. Furthermore, not mentioning smoking is often viewed by the smoker as passive endorsement by the GP of their smoking habit.

Smoking cessation guidelines for health professionals propose the '5 A's' approach to helping smokers to quit:

The 5 A's approach to helping smoking cessation

Ask all patients about their smoking history 'Have you ever tried to stop?'

Advise all patients to quit, using personalized but non-judgemental language — 'I think it is important for you to quit smoking and I can help you'

Assess motivation to quit 'How do you feel about smoking? Are you ready to give up?'

Assist motivated smokers by giving further advice and prescribing nicotine replacement therapy or Buproprion — Based on readiness to quit. For smokers who are ready, a quit plan is helpful:
- *Set a quit date.*
- *Tell family, friends and co-workers about quitting and request understanding and support*
- *Anticipate challenges to planned quit attempt*
- *Remove tobacco products from the environment.*

Arrange appropriate follow-up — For those who are ready, the local smoking cessation services are the most effective referral route.

Brief interventions for alcohol

It is estimated that one third of British men and one fifth of women drink more than the 'safe' alcohol levels recommended in the 'Health of the Nation' targets. Brief alcohol interventions aim to reduce long-term alcohol use and related harm in individuals attending primary care facilities but not seeking help for alcohol-related problems. Studies have found they are effective in reducing alcohol consumption at 6 and 12 months by an average of nearly five units a week (a unit of alcohol is a drink containing 8 g of ethanol – the equivalent of half a pint of 3.5% proof beer, or a single measure of spirits; a 125 ml glass of 12% wine is 1.5 units). While the exact format for a brief intervention for alcohol is not as clearly defined as it is for tobacco, an intervention usually includes:

- Assessment of intake.
- Provision of information and advice on 'safe' levels and harms.
- Identification of high-risk situations for drinking.
- Coping strategies for dealing with high-risk situations.
- Increasing motivation.
- Development of a personal plan to reduce drinking.

Other ways of categorizing health promotion

Degree of empowerment
Risk factors
Disease or condition
Settings and groups

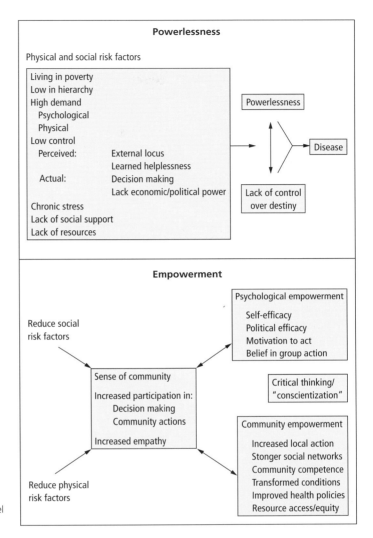

Figure 11.8 The empowerment model of health promotion.

Degrees of empowerment

The empowerment model of health promotion, looking beyond prevention, protection and health education alone to fostering improvements in material circumstances such as diet, housing, income and skills, through creating environments where personal and community empowerment, is allowed to flourish. Where people are powerless, for reasons of social and economic disadvantage defined as 'social and physical risk factors' in Figure 11.8, they lack control over their destiny and are more vulnerable to ill health and misfortune. Where these social and physical risk factors are reduced, as the lower part of Figure 11.8 indicates, self-efficacy and community-efficacy increase, leading to actions that will promote health.

Risk factors

Tobacco, alcohol and obesity are all acknowledged risk factors in health promotion, so working on these risk factors is health promoting in its own right.

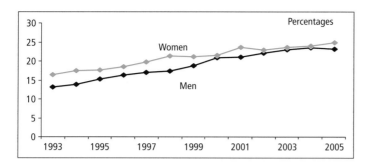

Figure 11.9 Obesity rates among adults in England, 1993–2005 (Source: Health Survey for England 2005: www.statistics.gov.uk).

Case study: Obesity as a public health problem

Obesity has been defined as 'a condition in which abnormal or excessive fat accumulation in adipose tissue impairs health'. The most widely used way of measuring it is the Body Mass Index (BMI). BMI represents weight (kg)/height (m)^2. In adults, obesity is regarded as a BMI of 30 or above. BMI in children is harder to calculate as it varies with age and sex. The measure can also be skewed in all ages by high muscle mass.

Obesity greatly increases the risk of type II diabetes and gall bladder disease. It is also a risk factor for heart disease, hypertension and stroke, as well as some cancers (e.g. colon, breast and endometrium). It is estimated that 10% of cancers affecting non-smokers are due to obesity.

In the early 1980s, 6% of men and 8% of women in the UK were obese. Obesity is increasing among both children and adults in the UK – it has gone up by just under 10% in both sexes over 12 years (Figure 11.10).

Obesity is unequally distributed globally. It is no longer a disease of purely affluent, developed countries. In 1995 it was estimated that worldwide there were 200 million obese adults and 18 million overweight children aged under five. By 2000, it was estimated there were over 300 million obese adults in the world of whom less than half (132 million) were in developed countries. Overall, the increase in the prevalence of obesity has been most dramatic among more affluent populations of less developed countries. Paradoxically, within affluent, developed countries obesity tends to be concentrated among those from lower income groups.

Figure 11.11 indicates the ways in which medicine – from public health medicine at the base, in the prevention arena, through primary and community care to hospital-based services – can be involved in dealing with what has come to be known as the obesity epidemic.

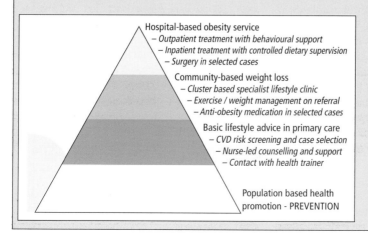

Figure 11.10 Ways of managing obesity in different settings (adapted with permission from Alan Maryon-Davies, 2004).

Population-based compared to individuals at risk-based interventions for obesity

Population	Individuals at risk
Advantages	*Advantages*
• Large numbers benefit • Lifestyle changes are modest and achievable • Different sectors and agencies can contribute • Relatively low cost	• Resources can be focused on those most likely to benefit • At-risk individuals may be more motivated to make lifestyle changes • It is easier to attribute effects to efforts • The evidence for effectiveness is stronger • Performance management systems can be set to encourage the adoption of the at-risk approach
Problems	*Problems*
• People are often resistant to changing their lifestyle • Main determinants are often beyond an individual's scope for control • The process may be very long-term	• Potential for victim-blaming • Individuals may feel stigmatized and experience negative body image • Weighing and measuring can be sensitive • One-to-one or group work is resource-intensive • Pressure on time allocated consultations may be inhibitory • Possibly language and cultural barriers

Tackling obesity requires a whole system approach involving partners from the NHS, local authorities, private sector, education, patient groups, voluntary and community sectors, regional and central government as well as multinational food enterprises.

Examples of programmes some Primary Care Trusts have developed in partnership with other organizations to help prevent and manage obesity include:

• 'Cook and eat' sessions for young people to encourage healthy eating behaviours, improve cookery skills and enhance confidence/self-esteem.
• '30 minutes active time' during normal working hours for all staff to encourage an activity of their choice.
• Working with local authorities to establish low-cost passes to leisure centre as incentives for employees.
• Regular lunchtime walks scheme.
• 'Step-o-meter' league and awards.

• 'Walking for health' groups using trained volunteer walk leaders and easy walks guides.
• 'Easy rides' cycle programmes providing information on short cycle rides along traffic-free and quiet roads in the area, along with adult cycle training schemes.
• Exercise on referral.
• Fruit and vegetables on prescription.
• Weight management referral schemes.
• Healthy lunchbox promotions.
• Free holiday exercise (e.g. swimming schemes).
• Buggy walks and Tumble Tots (physical play programmes for young children).
• Breastfeeding support and awareness.

Health promotion by disease or condition

Focusing on a particularly disease or condition enables targeted work on public health problems of concern.

Case study: Suicide prevention

Some common myths about suicide

Myth	Fact
Suicide is relatively rare	Suicide is one of the ten commonest causes of death, accounting for 5000 deaths per year in the UK, 1% of the total deaths.
Suicide is never a most common cause of death among any group	In 2002, suicide was the most common cause of death for men under 35
Suicides are 'loners'	Nearly two-thirds of those who commit suicide live with someone
Job stress is a common form of suicide	Although 40% of those who commit suicide are employed, the unemployed are three times more likely to kill themselves than people in employment
People who are considering suicide rarely talk to anyone about it	68% of people who commit suicide express ideas about it before they act
People who are seriously considering suicide rarely come into contact with the medical services	In the preceding three months 66% of suicide cases have seen a GP, and 25% of suicides are psychiatric out-patients
Scottish people are less likely to kill themselves than the English and Welsh	Scotland's suicide rate is twice that of England and Wales. It has increased by 70% over the last 30 years
The role of the police is only to assist post-mortem	A quarter of suicide cases have seen a police officer in the previous three months, half as a victim of crime
Women are more likely to kill themselves than men	Men are nearly three times more likely to kill themselves than women, across the age groups. Men tend to use more violent and lethal suicide methods (hanging and suffocation and poisoning by gases and vapour have both increased steadily since 1983)
Leaving a suicide note is common	Only one in six suicides leave a note

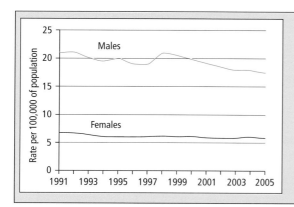

Figure 11.11 Suicide rates, England and Wales, by gender (Source: National Statistics website: www.statistics.gov.uk).

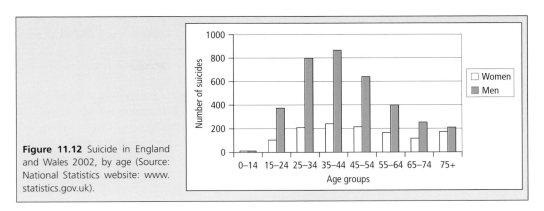

Figure 11.12 Suicide in England and Wales 2002, by age (Source: National Statistics website: www. statistics.gov.uk).

The National Service Framework wants health and social care services to play a full part in reducing the suicide rate by at least 20% by 2010.

What can an individual do to help reduce suicide rates?

Look for clues (euphemisms) in what people say, e.g.
– 'I wish I wasn't here'.
– 'I may be leaving soon'.
– 'I wish I could just go to sleep'.
– 'I'm no use to anyone anymore; it's just hopeless'.
– 'People would be better off without me'.
– 'I cannot cope with this illness'.
– 'I am too old for life'.

There is no evidence that mentioning suicide causes suicide
• In fact. it is more likely to reduce it as the person is being listened to, often for first time.

Don't be afraid to ask direct but tactful questions about suicide ideas, e.g.
– General mood questions.
– How do you see the future?
– Have you ever felt life isn't worth living?
– Have you ever wished you could go to sleep and not wake up?
– Have you ever thought of wanting to die? If so:
– Have you ever considered suicide? Have you thought how?

– What has stopped you so far?
– How do you cope when things get this bad?
– What do you think might make you go ahead?

Don't offer false reassurance ('Oh, you'll be OK'), but *help to solve the problem* ('What can we do to make this better?')
Don't avoid the word suicide e.g. by saying 'you know' or 'hurting yourself'.
Monitor your own feelings and attitudes.
Follow up 'not really' statements.
Go back to the topic again if necessary as rapport develops (e.g. if inconsistencies or true emotions come out later in interview).

Settings and groups for health promotion

Particular settings and population groups provide opportunities for health promotion that might otherwise be unavailable. A focus on particular setting enables health promotion work to be appropriate for the issues and concerns arising in that setting. It also enables a range of activities to be included under one umbrella such as 'healthy schools' or 'healthy cities'. Settings-based health promotion enables consideration of the issues faced by the specific group(s) of people found in that setting, and the development of messages and materials appropriate for them. Sometimes finding appropriate settings for work with hard-to-reach groups needs imagination. For example, injecting drug users may be assisted by health promotion materials in public toilets, if drugs and needles are known to be exchanged there. Sex workers may need to be targeted on the streets or in clubs and bars. Community and voluntary sector organizations may be the most appropriate way to work with groups such as ethnic minority populations, asylum seekers and refugees.

Much settings-based health promotion work takes place in the workplace, encouraged by employers who see it as a way of achieving fewer sickness absences and of enhancing their public profile as a 'healthy employer'. It should not be forgotten that hospitals, schools, prisons and other institutions dealing with particular groups of people are also workplaces and sites for work with other 'stakeholders'.

Examples of settings with diverse groups for health promotion

Setting	Group(s)
Schools	School children
	Teachers
	Ancillary and support staff
	Parents and communities
Prisons	Prisoners
	Staff
	Visitors
Universities/medical schools	Students
	Academic staff
	Ancillary and support staff
	Communities (through outreach)

Summary

- Health promotion can be subdivided into methods: disease prevention, health protection and health education.
- The empowerment model is another approach to health promotion.
- Health promotion can also focus on risk factors, disease or condition, settings and groups.
- There are many reasons for people to behave 'irrationally' and not follow 'healthy' behaviour patterns.

- The stages of change model can be applied to many habits and addictions as a tool to ascertain a person's readiness to change.
- Need is in the eye of the beholder, and may involve a hierarchy.
- There are many ways for doctors to be usefully involved in health promotion work, such as brief interventions for quitting smoking and reducing alcohol consumption, obesity management in primary and secondary care, and suicide prevention.
- Settings for health promotion work include institutions such as schools, prisons, hospitals and universities – these are also workplaces and visitor sites.

Further reading

Davison, C., Davey Smith, G. and Frankel, S. (1991) Lay epidemiology and the prevention paradox: the implications of coronary candidacy for health education. *Sociology of Health and Illness*, **13**(1): 1–19.

Farmer, R. and Lawrenson, R. (2004) *Lecture Notes: Epidemiology and Public Health Medicine* (5th edn.). Oxford: Blackwell, Part 2: Prevention and Control of Disease.

Maryon-Davis, A. (2004) Obesity Action Plan. Working Paper for the CHD NSF Implementation Group. London: Southwark Primary Care Trust.

Maryon-Davis, A. (2005) Weight management in primary care: How can it be made more effective? *Proceedings of the Nutrition Society*, **64**: 97–103.

Power, R. et al. (1999) Health, health promotion, and homelessness. *British Medical Journal*, **318**: 590–2.

Tones, K. and Green, J. (2004) *Health Promotion: Planning and Strategies*. London: Sage.

Wass, A. (2000) *Promoting Health: the Primary Health Care Approach*. Sydney: Harcourt-Saunders.

West, R., McNeill, A. and Raw, M. (2000) Smoking cessation guidelines for health professionals: an update. *Thorax*, **55**(12): 987–99.

Chapter 12

Chronic illness

Every living person has his own peculiarities and always has his own peculiar, personal, novel, complicated disease, unknown to medicine.

Leo Tolstoy, *War and Peace*

Introduction

An increasing number of the conditions dealt with by doctors today are long-term and chronic and can have a profound impact on the lives of their sufferers. Chronic illnesses challenge bio-medical models of care based on curative goals and require different skills on the part of doctors, since most of what doctors do for such people is palliative rather than curative. Understanding the experience of people with chronic health conditions is one way of arriving at a role which better serves the needs of the individuals concerned and the abilities of the medical profession to provide for them. It is important to work with the values, priorities and expectations of people who are chronically ill, as well as their families and carers, and to be aware of the services, such as self-help groups, that are available for them. Through such

Lecture Notes: The Social Basis of Medicine, 1st edition. By Andrew Russell. Published 2009 by Blackwell Publishing. ISBN: 978-1-4051-3912-0

a patient-centred approach, the welfare of people with chronic illnesses and the maintenance and improvement of the quality of their lives, rather than the eradication of the disease processes from which they are suffering, can become the doctor's priority.

> **This chapter covers the following topics**
>
> Chronic illness – a growing health concern
> The experience of people with chronic conditions
> Caring for people with chronic illness

Chronic illness – a growing health concern

What is chronic illness?

A chronic illness is any disease or disorder that continues over an extended period and causes continuous or episodic periods of incapacity. This definition covers a wide range of conditions that can affect almost all body systems.

Examples of chronic illnesses in the UK

- *Alzheimer's disease/Dementia.* Alzheimer's disease affects about 417,000 people and is the most common form of dementia.
- *Asthma* affects over 3.4 million people in the UK, including 1.5 million children aged 2–15.
- *Backache* of over a day's duration is self-reported by 40% of adults, of whom 15% say they are in constant pain.
- *Cancer.* There were about 2 million cancer survivors in 2008. This figure is increasing at the rate of 3.2% a year.
- *Chronic obstructive pulmonary disease (COPD).* Prevalence is uncertain.
- *Cystic fibrosis.* Incidence at birth is 1 in 2400.
- *Depression.* Lifetime risk for major depression is 15%–19% for women; 10% for men.
- *Diabetes mellitus* (Types I and II). Approximately 1.5 million diagnosed cases.
- *Eczema* affects 15–20% of school children and 2–10% of adults.
- *End-stage renal disease.* Approximately 100 per million reach end-stage renal failure each year and 600–800 per million rely on dialysis or transplant for survival.
- *Endometriosis.* Prevalence is uncertain – 2–22 per 1000 in asymptomatic women.
- *Epilepsy* affects more than 420,000 people, or 1 in 130 of the population.
- *Glaucoma* affects more than 2.2 million
- *Hearing impairment.* Prevalence of almost one in seven.
- *Heart failure* affects more than 500,000 people.
- *HIV/AIDS.* Approximately 73,000 are living with HIV.
- *Incontinence* affects 5–9% of the total population.
- *Leprosy* (Hansen's disease). Rare.
- *Migraine* intermittently affects 8 million people.
- *Multiple sclerosis* affects 80,000–90,000 people.
- *Parkinson's disease* affects 120,000 people.
- *Poliomyelitis.* Now all but eradicated in the UK.
- *Psoriasis* has a prevalence of 2%.
- *Rheumatoid arthritis* affects about 8.5 million people, of whom 14,500 are children.
- *Schizophrenia.* Prevalence of 3.4 per 1000 adults a year.
- *Stroke* affects 5.18 per 1000.
- *Ulcerative* colitis affects 80 per 100,000.

The symptomatology of these illnesses varies dramatically between illnesses and among sufferers of the same illness. Advances in medical treatment have changed the status of some illnesses from acute to chronic. One example is the development of anti-retroviral drugs for HIV/AIDS, which have transformed what was previously almost invariably a fatal disease into a chronic health condition. The prognosis for different kinds of cancer has also changed and in most cases has improved.

Prevalence of chronic illness

One in three (roughly 17 million people) UK adults report a long-standing illness, with one in

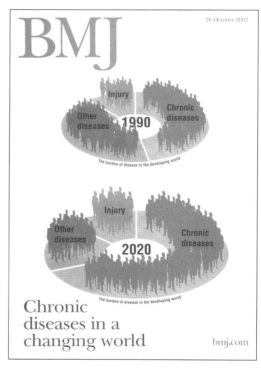

Figure 12.1 Front cover of the *British Medical Journal*, **332**, 26 October 2002 (reproduced with permission of the BMJ Publishing Group).

Table 12.1 Prevalence of chronic health problems in the UK (Source: British Household Panel survey, 2001: www. statistics.gov.uk).

Chronic problem	No (%) of respondents (n = 5500) reporting in 2001
High prevalence	
None	2129 (38.7)
Problems or disability connected with: arms, legs, hands, feet, back, or neck (including arthritis and rheumatism)	1639 (28.0)
Heart problems, high blood pressure or blood circulation problems	924 (16.8)
Middling prevalence	
Chest or breathing problems, asthma, bronchitis	743 (13.5)
Skin conditions or allergies	616 (11.2)
Anxiety, depression or bad nerves, psychiatric problems	490 (8.9)
Stomach, liver, kidney or digestive problems	468 (8.5)
Difficulty in hearing	435 (7.9)
Migraine or frequent headaches	435 (7.9)
Low prevalence	
Difficulty in seeing (other than needing glasses to read normal-size print)	281 (5.1)
Stroke	220 (4.0)
Diabetes	193 (3.5)
Other health problems	83 (1.5)
Cancer	77 (1.4)
Epilepsy	50 (0.9)
Alcohol or drug-related problems	33 (0.6)

five having something serious enough that it causes them to cut down on their activities. The British Household Panel is an ongoing survey of some 5500 households which includes questions about prevalence of chronic health problems (Table 12.1). The commonest reported problems are those of the cardiovascular and musculoskeletal systems.

The prevalence of chronic illness is increasing worldwide. Figure 12.1 demonstrates graphically how the burden of disease in the developing world is also shifting from acute to chronic conditions.

Age and chronic illness – a demographic time-bomb?

Figure 12.2 shows the dramatic increase in life expectancy at birth in the past 100 years. Chronic illness increases with an ageing population, since it is particularly associated with the elderly. For example, in a survey conducted in 1998, 80% of

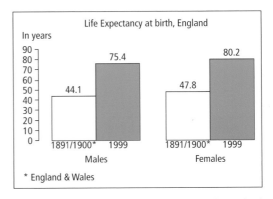

Figure 12.2 Change in life expectancy at birth, England and Wales.

Americans aged over 65 reported suffering from at least one chronic illness. However, it should not be forgotten that children may also be affected by chronic illnesses. In the UK, 15% of under-fives and 20% aged 5–15 are said to have a long-term health condition.

Projected changes for the UK population

Figure 12.3 shows the predicted population changes for all age groups compared to the age groups 65–79 and 80+ from an index of 100 in 2001 for each group. In 2001, it is estimated there were 6.9 million people aged 65–79 (12% of the population), with 2.5 million (4%) aged 80 or more. By 2051, based on 2004 projections, 25% of the population will be over 65, of whom two-thirds will be over 80. The total population is predicted to rise more gradually, from 59.1 million in 2001 to 69.3 million in 2051. However, while increasing life expectancy will result in many more old people living in Britain, it is not clear that life expectancy free of illness will increase at the same rate. In other words, the burden of chronic illness is likely to increase.

At present, people suffering from chronic health conditions constitute 80% of all GP consultations. Moreover, someone with a chronic health condition is at least twice as likely to be admitted as an inpatient for a particular condition compared to someone without one, and will spend longer in hospital. The health care costs of dealing with chronic health conditions increase dramatically over the life span.

The situation in the US (see Figure 12.4) is similar to that found in the UK. Although the overall health profile of the population has improved dramatically and most people now live a long, healthy life, with only intermittent problems or chronic conditions which remain compatible with a reasonable quality of life (allowing for the inequalities in health discussed in Chapter 7), problems tend to cluster in the final years of life, which are marked by increasingly fragile health and complex care needs.

Inequalities in chronic illness

Chronic illness, like illness in general (Chapter 7), is not randomly distributed in the population. As well as the rates of chronic illness increasing substantially with age, they are also higher among women and tend to be class-related (Figure 12.5).

Chronic illnesses pose risks that are common to all sufferers, regardless of the condition they have. All of these can have knock-on effects on health and well-being, which in turn may contribute to further downward social mobility.

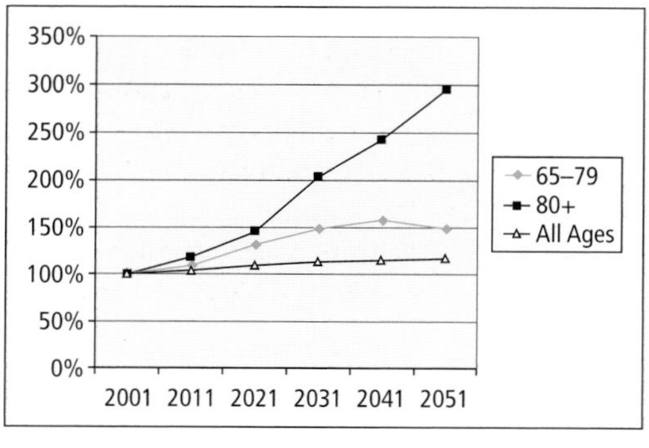

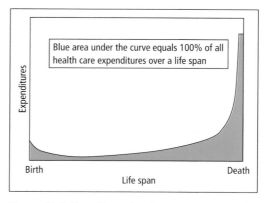

Figure 12.3 Projected population changes by age groups, 2004 (Government Actuary's Department, www.statistics.gov.uk).

Figure 12.4 Chart illustrating how Americans' health care expenditures are concentrated in the final stages of life (Reproduced with permission of the Rand Corporation).

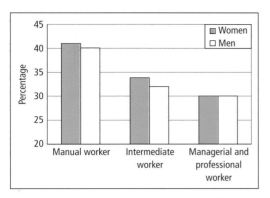

Figure 12.5 Percentage of General Household Survey 2002 respondents (n = 13,000) reporting a longstanding health problem (Source: Wilson et al., 2005).

Factors that explain patient delay

Illness – nature of symptoms; how soon they are noticeable.
Appraisal – self-diagnosis of symptoms' significance (affected by knowledge of symptoms).
Behavioural delay – fear (e.g. of cancer, HIV/AIDS); chaotic lifestyle.
Scheduling delay – lack of time to arrange/attend an appointment.
Personal reticence/lack of assertiveness.

Common risks with chronic illness

- Unemployment or underemployment.
- Reduced career prospects.
- Social isolation.
- Loss or change of important roles.
- Changed physical appearance.
- Problems with self-esteem and identity.

The experience of people with chronic conditions

Common themes in the experience of people with chronic conditions

- Uncertainty.
- Stigma.
- Biographical work/reconstitution of self.
- Managing regimens.
- Communication and support.
- Family relationships.

Uncertainty

Uncertainty is a problem both pre- and post-diagnosis. Many patients with chronic health conditions wait a long time before their problem is properly diagnosed (though this may be due to patient delay, as is often the case with rectal bleeding).

However, presenting with a complaint does not mean that diagnosis will be automatic, particularly where a disease is rare, the symptoms are non-specific or the course of the illness is unusual in any way. Sometimes the delay in diagnosis can be considerable. The average length of time for people suffering from ankylosing spondylitis to receive a diagnosis, for example, is over eight years. In one study of 30 people suffering from multiple sclerosis the delay in diagnosis was up to 15 years.

Post-diagnosis uncertainty may be long-term or short-term. Long-term, there is uncertainty as to how the person is likely to end up and on what timescale. Short-term are the day-to-day symptom fluctuations, a particular problem for those with rheumatoid arthritis.

Uncertainty makes planning difficult and may require constant revision of living arrangements.

Stigma

The duration of many chronic illnesses means that a sense of stigma (Chapter 2) can be particularly profound.

Four characteristics affecting the extent to which a chronic disease is likely to be stigmatized

1 When the cause of a condition is perceived (rightly or wrongly) to be the bearer's responsibility.
2 When a condition is perceived as unalterable or degenerative.
3 When conditions are perceived as contagious or to place others in danger.
4 When a condition is readily apparent to others and is perceived as repellent, ugly or upsetting (e.g. if it creates discomfort in social settings).

There is evidence that many people with chronic illnesses use coping strategies such as secrecy and withdrawal to deal with the perceived likelihood of discrimination against them. Thus stigma is perpetuated not only by its enactment (direct and indirect discriminatory behaviour by others) but also through the perceptions and expectations of those suffering from the illness. Stigma may be quite irrational, as in the case of epilepsy (see below).

Case study: epilepsy as a stigmatized condition

Epilepsy is an extremely variable disease, but is generally a benign disorder with an excellent clinical prognosis except for the 20–30% of people whose seizures do not respond to treatment and tend to be associated with high levels of psychiatric comorbidity and low quality of life.

However, the social prognosis of epilepsy tends to be less rosy than the clinical one. Epilepsy exhibits all the characteristics of a highly stigmatized disease, particularly in countries lacking the health resources for its adequate treatment and for those in wealthier countries with intractable seizures. Reasons for this may include:

- Onlookers fear the symptoms and may feel endangered by someone in seizure (i.e. symptoms cause discomfort in social situations).
- Seizure timings are unpredictable and the sufferer appears 'out of control'.
- People do not know how to deal with the symptoms and hence feel impotent.
- Epilepsy may (wrongly) be considered a mental rather than a physical illness.
- Other imperfections are attributed to people with epilepsy, e.g. that they are potentially violent, retarded, weak, sluggish, slow, antisocial and unattractive.
- Seizures are difficult to conceal, disruptive and sometimes aesthetically unpleasant.
- The cause of epilepsy is uncertain (congenital, accidental or intentional).

Because seizures tend to be irregular and transient, epilepsy is more frequently discreditable than discrediting (see Chapter 2). Controlling the information about their discreditable and potentially discrediting ailment can cause sufferers considerable amounts of 'hidden distress' as they seek to avoid enacted stigma. A sense of stigma persists for some people even when their seizures are well controlled, and can be enacted in the fields of education, employment, insurance and health care provision. Studies have indicated that the 'felt stigma' (e.g. the feeling that having epilepsy is a disadvantage in the job market) may be much more widespread than 'enacted stigma' (e.g. the ability to attribute specific employment problems to having epilepsy), although in job recruitment the existence of prejudicial views may be difficult to prove.

Biographical work/reconstitution of self

Illness is always a disruptive event. When it is clear that it is not self-limiting or cured this leads to changes in an individual's perception of themselves and their position in society. The assumption of many (not necessarily all) that their life will be reasonably long and healthy is unexpectedly challenged: a degree of control has been lost. Chronically ill people may struggle to lead valued lives and to maintain images of themselves as someone with a life that is worthwhile.

As part of the process of coming to terms with their illness, people undergo a process of 'narrative reconstruction', invoking lay (and sometimes medical) theories of illness aetiology and other explanations in order to regain a sense of meaning and structure that the illness may have taken away from them.

Case study: Am I still me?

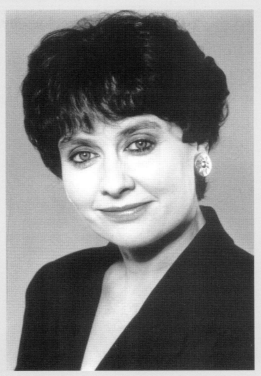

In 1999 the broadcaster Sheena McDonald suffered a major road traffic injury. She writes:

'I was hit by a police van while I was crossing the road on 26 February 1999. It was late at night and raining. The van was travelling on the wrong side of the road. I remember nothing about what happened to me. I was taken by ambulance to the nearest hospital's Accident and Emergency Unit. Intubation was carried out to allow assisted ventilation because I couldn't breathe for myself. I had suffered such a severe head injury that the medical profession thought that surviving at all was as much as could be expected. Just over a year after the injury, a doctor described me as 'a walking miracle' – and I was still in primary recovery. I suffered five or six weeks of what's called post-traumatic amnesia. Conventional neurological wisdom insists that such a period of amnesia inevitably changes the sufferer. I was so determined to recover fully that I found it impossible to believe that I would be changed as a result – that I would somehow not be fully 'me' any more.

  Five years on, I'm very much better. My mother says she always knew I would recover, and would mutter 'Get a grip, Sheena!' to my hospital bed – so I joke that I didn't dare not recover for fear of disobeying her. Given that the professionals are surprised – to the best of my knowledge, 'miracle' is not a clinical term – I now have a layman's obsession to understand as much as I can about how the brain works – and how mine defied convention. Doctors used to think recovery stops after a few months, but I'm living proof that this is not so. Conventional wisdom may be based on the kind of people who normally suffer my injury – young men on drink or drugs without fully developed brains or long-term stimulating care and support. Of course, given the nature of my condition, my claimed expertise and authority on having been through serious trauma is tempered by the practical reality of being traumatised. What did happen to me? What makes me me? And am I the same 'me' I was five years ago? I am convinced that I am myself, and those bold enough to hire me to do what I used to do – work as a broadcast journalist – seem satisfied that this person called Sheena McDonald is as good as ever. But am I a cunning simulation of the person I was? Or will I achieve lasting fame as a neurological footnote for freakishness? Or even change what neuroscientists expect of the severely head-injured?'

Managing regimens

The person with a chronic illness needs to engage in two sorts of management regimen – the management of their life to take into account the limitations and control imposed by their symptoms, and the management of the medical regimens designed to limit and control those symptoms.

A person with rheumatoid arthritis needs to arrange their life around the symptoms by deciding how much activity is possible or likely before too much pain sets in and they have to rest.

Medical regimens may include diet, drugs or the use of advanced technologies such as a kidney dialysis machine. Somebody who is HIV-positive, for example, can be taking up to 10 pharmaceutical products per day. Managing medical regimens involves time, energy and financial resources. Such activities have been called 'illness work'. Over and above the problems of the illness itself, such medical regimens can affect someone's ability to perform paid work. In extreme circumstances the whole life of the chronically ill person can be organized around treatment (see below). Sometimes the sufferer will alter their prescribed regimen. This gives them the chance to exert some degree of control over their illness and so avoid some of the more negative aspects of the treatments it requires.

Case study: Life with 'Fifi', a Cape Cuirass ventilator

David Brooks was an anthropology lecturer. In 1991 he wrote:

'It was August 1989 when I first connected to Fifi, my Cape Cuirass pump. The pair of us are joined in mock matrimony by a length of black hosepipe. Fifi huffs and puffs away all night long while I sleep, content in the knowledge that she will take sole care of the business of breathing. We have been sleeping together for about six months. When I was first introduced to Fifi, I did not believe I could ever get used to the noisy machine and the fancy dress. However, just one night converted me to the joys and thrills of home ventilation.

In the autumn on 1966 I was involved in a car accident while a research student in Iran. My injuries included a fractured pelvis, a badly torn diaphragm and ruptured spleen. Life went on. Twenty years later, a growing breathlessness was eventually diagnosed as lung cancer. The malignancy affected my right lung only, not the left one, damaged in the car accident. It was decided, in spite of the denervated diaphragm, that I ought to be able to cope with the left lung alone. In December 1986 a right pneumonectomy was performed and invaded lymph nodes removed. December 1988 saw me bedridden again. By April I was taken into hospital once more. This time no signs of cancer were found. I continued to lose weight, in part because I could not eat easily. Chewing food was exhausting, even swallowing liquids was difficult. I had lost my grip and had started to drop things from my grasp. I could scarcely walk. I felt totally drained of energy and kept falling asleep. I had developed frequent, odd headaches. Most disturbingly my thought processes had lost coherence.

I was referred back to hospital in mid-July. A 'sleep study' was performed and, like magic, literally overnight the source of my symptoms lay revealed, the denervated diaphragm, a legacy of the past. I repeatedly stopped breathing while I slept. I was being oxygen starved and carbon dioxide levels sent askew. The diagnosis, with the prospect of helpful night-time ventilation, came when it did as a most welcome, life-saving relief, in total contrast to the initial desolation following the previous diagnosis of lung cancer. That the Cape Cuirass Pump was a non-invasive machine was an added bonus. I was first tried on a nasal IPPV machine. This system, however, painfully inflated my stomach rather than my lung, and the mask resulted in excessive salivation. The negative pressure ventilation system produced no such problems. I managed to sleep reasonably well, and the virtually instant amelioration of at least some of my symptoms had me almost euphoric, the consequence of an exhilarating heightening of my dulled sensory perception. An overall sense of well-being accompanied a renewed visual, aural and tactile sensitivity. Ten days later I returned home happily with Fifi. My breathlessness remains chronic, but Fifi has undoubtedly enhanced the quality of my life.

Within a few weeks I was used again to feeling alert and settled down to my long-term affair with Fifi. Almost inevitably I fell into the luxury of thinking that the major turnaround in my health, brought about by home ventilation, meant I would 'get well again', that I would somehow recover, the way one does from illnesses. Fifi, of course, is an aid, not a cure. There is no 'cure' for one lung and a dead diaphragm.

After a busy day in the armchair, I retire, hot with fatigue, struggle impatiently into the ventilation jacket and breathlessly but gratefully attach myself to Fifi. I have become quite shamelessly addicted to her ministrations, since only then does the exhaustion of breathing for myself fade away, the aches and pains of the day dissolve and the always lurking claustrophobia disappear. Although I am enormously restricted physically, Fifi has made possible a return to a life that was ebbing away a year before, a return to an albeit altered participation in family life, and even to writing a bit again.'

David Brooks died in 1994.

Information, communication and support

Information and communication issues are crucial for people with chronic health conditions because so much is dependent on quality of life. Information is vital for the chronically ill and their carers, in order to reduce uncertainty, to help them come to terms with the illness and the altered person it creates, and for the development of ways of managing the illness as best they can.

It may be difficult for patients with chronic health conditions to communicate straightforwardly. Chronic illness etiquette, the sense that people get tired of hearing about their problems, may lead to people 'masking' their symptoms. Some conditions, such as the 'expressive mask' of Parkinson's disease, may lead to inadvertent problems with non-verbal communication. Finally, exclusion of the patient's perspective as an irrelevance or a nuisance in consultations with the chronically ill can lead to a sense of voicelessness which may be exacerbated by pain, depression or mental confusion. (Voicelessness is also a problem for people for whom English is not a first language, whether or not they are suffering from a chronic health condition.)

Clearly the structure of many medical consultations (e.g. restricted time slots and less continuity of care) does not necessarily facilitate the 'patient-centred' consultations that are necessary in order for the whole-person approach to be successful (Chapter 6). People with chronic illnesses frequently spend only a fraction of their time in a patient ('sick') role, but much of their time being ill. It is therefore likely that they have many ideas and concerns that they bring to the clinical encounter which cannot always be addressed. Self-help groups (see Chapter 3) have an important part to play in supporting patients and their families, and redressing some of the inadequacies of clinical service delivery for the chronically ill.

Case study: The NHS Expert Patient Programme

The Expert Patient Programme (EPP) was established in 2002 as a training programme to enable people living with chronic conditions to become equal partners with their health professionals, and to develop skills such as action planning and problem-solving that would enable them to take over some of the management of their illness. It is based on a similar programme developed in Stanford, California. At the local level a network of trainers and about 1400 tutors with long-term conditions lead the EPP. Participation is voluntary and all the tutors are volunteers. The training centres on a six-week course comprising weekly sessions 2½ hours long which aim to give patients the skills necessary to improve their quality of life. There are also 'Looking After Me' courses for carers of people suffering from chronic health conditions. Online versions have been developed for people living in remote areas or who are unable to attend sessions in their local community.

Five core self-management skills have been identified and these are the focus of the programme:

1 Problem-solving.
2 Decision-making.

(continued on p. 172)

(continued)

3 Resource utilization.
4 Developing effective partnerships with health care providers.
5 Taking action.
Specific areas of the programme involve developing:

- Communication skills.
- Interaction with the health care system.
- Finding health resources.
- Planning for the future.
- Understanding exercise and healthy eating.
- Management of feelings and emotions (e.g. fatigue, sleep, pain, anger and depression).

Some courses are run for people with specific health conditions, others for people with more general problems (e.g. people at risk of falls), while yet others are for people suffering from any chronic condition. Some doctors dislike the term 'expert patient'; they find it confrontational and would prefer 'involved patient'.

In 2007, the programme became the first national community interest company in the UK, the Expert Patient Programme CIC. This is a new way of enabling the sustainability of initiatives such as this through the development of not-for-profit companies.

Does it work?

About 20,000 people took the programme in its first five years. Courses cost about £300 per person but are free at point of delivery. A randomized controlled evaluation was carried out of 629 patients who were either given an EPP course or put on a six-month waiting list for a course. Contrary to predictions, there was no change in health services utilization (i.e. the number of GP consultations, practice nurse appointments, A&E attendances and outpatient visits); however, overnight hospital stays and use of day-care facilities were reduced in the EPP group. This means that, on balance, the programme is likely to be cost-effective. More telling were the patients' experience of EPP: subjective and objective measures indicated they were very satisfied with the course and the small gains in their energy levels they reported. There were also improvements in their quality of life and their ability to manage their condition. The courses tended to reinforce the value of patients' existing self-care activities rather than initiating new behaviours. There was a relatively low recognition of the initiative among the health and social care community, with GPs and health professionals generally slow to engage with the programme. The conclusion was that the EPP, rather than a panacea, is a useful adjunct to current services for some individuals. As it is voluntary, the results are only applicable to those who volunteer, not to the total population of chronic illness sufferers.

The course may have more to offer those whose needs are only met in a limited way by existing services (e.g. those with 'uncertain conditions') rather than those who are already 'well plugged in' to existing forms of service use. There is also scope for greater integration of self-management programmes within existing health care provision rather than as separate, community-led initiatives.

Family relationships

Aspects of family relationships potentially affected by chronic illness

Care and support
Emotions of giving and receiving care
Changes in family roles and relationships
Sexual capacity
Withdrawing (e.g. as a result of pain)
Social isolation

It is estimated that approximately 95% of informal care (i.e. unpaid care, predominantly to family members, neighbours and relatives) is provided in the family, much of it by women. It is estimated that if all the informal care that is provided to sick people in the UK were paid for out of the public purse, the total expenditure would be between £15 billion and £24 billion. The peak age for becoming a carer is 45–64, with approximately 20% of people in this age group providing some kind of informal care.

Informal carers provide unpaid care for family members, friends, neighbours or others who are sick, disabled or elderly. In April 2001 there were 5.9 million informal carers in the UK of whom the majority were women (3. 4 million compared with 2.5 million men). Around a quarter of both male and female carers were aged 45–54 with around a fifth falling in each of the adjacent age groups (35–44 and 55–64). A fifth of all carers were caring for 50 hours a week or more; two-thirds were caring for less than 20 hours per week. Women were slightly more likely than men to be caring for 50 hours or more, while men were slightly more likely than women to be caring for less than 20 hours. However, for those aged 85 and over, male carers were more likely than female carers to be caring for 50 hours or more (54 per cent compared with 47 per cent).

In 2001 there were 179,000 male carers and 169,000 female carers aged 75 and over – 12 per cent of men in this age group and 7 per cent of women. Owing to the relative longevity of the sexes, older women are more likely to be widowed and hence are more likely to be living alone and receiving care from personal social services and less likely to be providing care to a spouse. In the UK, although there was little difference between the proportions of men and women receiving home help in most age groups, a greater of proportion of women than men aged 85 and over received private or local authority home help in 2001/2.

The emotions involved in giving and receiving informal care can be complex – generosity and resentment in the mind of the giver, gratitude and resentment in the mind of the recipient. This is particularly the case where conventional roles (e.g. male breadwinner, female nurturer/carer) are overturned as a result of chronic illness.

Sexual capacity may be inhibited either through the illness itself (e.g. impotence with diabetes) or through embarrassment at the outcomes of the illness (e.g. a stoma bag following a colostomy for rectal cancer). Many doctors refrain from asking a patient about their sex life for fear of embarrassment, but it is often the most distressing aspect of a chronic illness. Like domestic violence (see Chapter 3), it is certainly worth asking about. Other symptoms and outcomes can cause an individual to withdraw from family life altogether (e.g. because of pain). Both individual and family can become isolated from the world around them.

Caring for people with chronic conditions

Different kinds of chronic conditions in the elderly can be categorized according to their likely 'trajectories':

Types of chronic conditions and their 'illness trajectories'

Non-fatal chronic illness	Rheumatoid arthritis Hearing and visual impairment
Serious, eventually fatal chronic conditions	Cancers Organ system failures (e.g. heart, liver, kidney, respiratory system) Dementia Stroke
Frailty	Few reserves leading to cascading health problems

Non-fatal chronic illnesses gradually worsen but seldom pose a direct threat to life. They may, however, cause considerable disability (see Chapter 10) and health care costs. The more serious conditions tend to worsen and are eventually fatal. Ninety per cent of elderly people have one or more of these conditions in the final years of their life. Frailty is seldom recognized as a disease category, but is a major feature of many elderly people's final years. The body's usual reserves diminish with age, and disease and small upsets are increasingly likely to lead to cascading health problems. Frailty is thus a serious health problem.

A short period of evident decline (upper part of Figure 12.6) is typical of cancer. Most people with cancer maintain their functioning and comfort for a considerable period, before declining quite rapidly in the final weeks/days before death when the illness becomes overwhelming. Hospice care

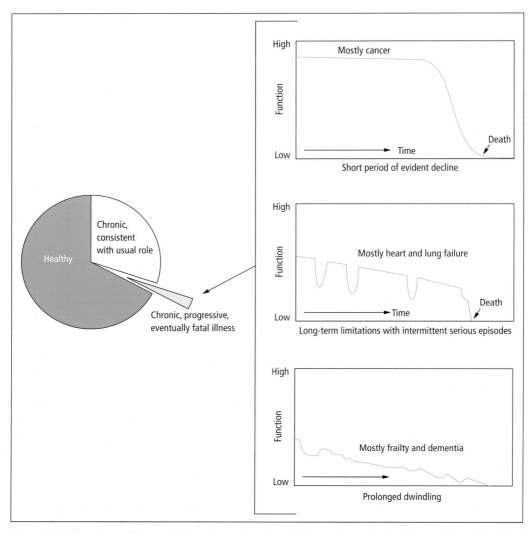

Figure 12.6 Three types of illness trajectory for serious chronic illnesses (Reproduced with permission of the Rand Corporation).

can be an important element of care for this trajectory. Long-term limitations with intermittent exacerbations and sudden death are typical of organ system failure (middle part of Figure 12.6). Ongoing disease management, advance care planning and home care services are important in this trajectory. Prolonged dwindling (lower part of Figure 12.6) is characteristic of frailty, disabling stroke and dementia. Again, home care services,

but followed up by institutional long-term care facilities, are important for this group.

The transition model (upper part of Figure 12.7) was based on aggressive, reactive care according to acute illness care models until the point when 'no more could be done' and the patient was regarded as 'terminally ill' and would ideally make a rapid transition into hospice care. However, the majority of chronically ill elderly patients

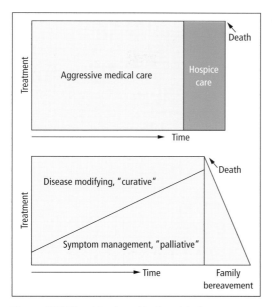

Figure 12.7 The older, 'transition' model of care versus a 'trajectory' model (Reproduced with permission of the Rand Corporation).

have an uncertain prognosis. For them, an abrupt transition from 'curative' to 'palliative' care is inappropriate – they continue to need a mix of patient-centred care, with a combination of treatments to stall the progression of their illness, relieve symptoms and provide support. This 'trajectory' model of care (lower part of Figure 12.7) also emphasizes the importance of supporting family members beyond the point of death (e.g. through bereavement counselling), although good hospice care also provides such support.

The National Service Framework for long-term conditions

In 2005, the NHS introduced a ten-year National Service Framework (NSF) for long-term conditions. Although it focuses on people with long-term neurological conditions, the NSF makes the point that much of the guidance offered can apply to anyone living with a long-term condition. Its 11 quality requirements are intended to transform the way health and social care services support people with long-term neurological conditions,

with the aim of allowing them to live as independently as possible.

The 11 requirements are as follows:

1 *Person-centred service:* People with long-term neurological conditions are to be offered integrated assessment and planning of their health and social care needs. They are to have the information they need to make informed decisions about their care and treatment and, where appropriate, to support them to manage their condition themselves.

2 *Early recognition, prompt diagnosis and treatment:* People suspected of having a neurological condition are to have prompt access to specialist neurological expertise for an accurate diagnosis, and treatment as close to home as possible.

3 *Emergency and acute management:* People needing hospital admission for a neurosurgical or neurological emergency are to be assessed and treated in a timely manner by teams with the appropriate neurological and resuscitation skills and facilities.

4 *Early and specialist rehabilitation:* People with long-term neurological conditions who would benefit from rehabilitation are to receive timely, ongoing, high-quality rehabilitation services in hospital or other specialist setting to meet their continuing and changing needs. When ready, they are to receive the help they need to return home for ongoing community rehabilitation and support.

5 *Community rehabilitation and support:* People with long-term neurological conditions living at home are to have ongoing access to a comprehensive range of rehabilitation, advice and support to meet their continuing and changing needs, increase their independence and autonomy, and help them to live as they wish.

6 *Vocational rehabilitation:* People with long-term neurological conditions are to have access to appropriate vocational assessment, rehabilitation and ongoing support to enable them to find, regain or remain in work and access other occupational and educational opportunities.

7 *Providing equipment and accommodation:* People with long-term neurological conditions are to receive timely, appropriate assistive technology/

equipment and adaptations to accommodation to support them to live independently, help them with their care, maintain their health and improve their quality of life.

8 *Providing personal care and support:* Health and social care services work together to provide care and support to enable people with long-term neurological conditions to achieve maximum choice about living independently at home.

9 *Palliative care:* People in the later stages of long-term neurological conditions are to receive a comprehensive range of palliative care services when they need them to control symptoms; offer pain relief and meet their needs for personal, social, psychological and spiritual support, in line with the principles of palliative care.

10 *Supporting family and carers:* Carers of people with long-term neurological conditions are to have access to appropriate support and services that recognize their needs both in their role as carer and in their own right.

11 *Caring for people with neurological conditions in hospital or other health and social care settings:* People with long-term neurological conditions are to have their specific neurological needs met while receiving care for other reasons in any health or social care setting.

There is little evidence that these requirements have improved the experience or outcomes of patients with chronic health conditions. Indeed, many believe crucial areas of care are suffering in the target-driven culture of today's NHS.

Summary

• People who are chronically ill spend only a small proportion of their time as a patient.

• Chronic illness challenges assumptions of medical care based on acute models.

• With an ageing population in the UK, chronic illness is likely to increase in the future.

• Chronic illness leads to uncertainty for patients and their families/carers.

• Some chronic illnesses are heavily stigmatized.

• Chronic illness may be the cause of considerable disruption to people's lives, expectations and sense of identity.

• Managing the regimens imposed by symptoms and medical treatments can be very difficult.

• Chronic illness can impose serious pressure on families and family relationships.

• The illness trajectories of elderly people with chronic health conditions varies and affects the type of care that may be most appropriate.

• The EPP and NSF for long-term conditions are attempts to improve the way in which people with chronic health conditions are dealt with by the NHS, although evidence for their effectiveness is patchy.

Further reading

Anderson, R. and Bury, M. (eds) (1988) *Living with Chronic Illness: the Experience of Patients and Their Families*. London: Unwin Hyman.

Brooks, D. H. M. (1992) Living with ventilation: confessions of an addict. *Care of the Critically Ill,* **8(5)**: 205–7.

Bury, M. (1997) *Health and Illness in a Changing Society*. London: Routledge, Chapter 4: Chronic illness and disability.

Conrad, P. (1990) Qualitative research on chronic illness: a commentary on methods and conceptual development. *Social Science and Medicine*, **30(1)**: 1257–63.

Crosland, A. and Jones, R. (1995) Rectal bleeding: prevalence and consultation behaviour. *British Medical Journal*, **311**: 486–8.

Greenhalgh, T. and Hurwitz, B. (1998) (eds) *Narrative Medicine: Dialogue and Discourse in Clinical Practice*. London: BMJ Books.

Jacoby, A., D. Snape and G. Baker (2005) Epilepsy and social identity: the stigma of a chronic neurological disorder. *Lancet Neurology*, **4**: 171–8.

Kleinman, A. (1988) *The Illness Narratives: Suffering, Healing and the Human Condition*. New York: Basic Books.

Kuh, D. and Ben-Shloms, Y. (eds) (1997) *A Life Course Approach to Chronic Disease Epidemiology*. Oxford: Oxford University Press.

Lewis, R. and Dixon, J. (2004) Rethinking management of chronic diseases. *British Medical Journal*, **328** (24 January): 220–2.

Locker, D. (2003) Living with chronic illness. In G. Scambler (ed.) *Sociology as Applied to Medicine* (5th edn.). Edinburgh: Saunders.

Lynn, J. and Adamson, D. M. (2003) *Living Well at the End of Life: Adapting Health Care to Serious Chronic Illness in Old Age*. Santa Monica, CA: Rand Health. http://www.rand.org/publications/WP/WP137/

Radley, A. (1993) The role of metaphor in adjustment to chronic illness. In A. Radley (ed.) *Worlds of Illness*. London: Routledge, pp 109–23.

Tickle-Degnen, L, and Doyle Lyons, K. (2004) Practitioners' impressions of patients with Parkinson's disease: the social ecology of the expressive mask. *Social Science and Medicine,* **58**: 603–14.

Wilson, T., Buck, D. and Ham, C. (2005) Rising to the challenge: will the NHS support people with long-term conditions? *British Medical Journal* **330**: 657–61.

Chapter 13

Death and dying

Introduction

Points of view

Imagine you were told you only had 3–6 months to live. How would this affect your life? What are the feelings you would be likely to experience? How would the knowledge you were terminally ill affect your priorities? How would it affect your family?

In confronting death, we confront the roots of our humanity. We can avoid many things, but death, 'the great leveller', comes to everyone. Some argue that without death, the pleasures and pains of life would have no meaning. But how we die, the management of dying and responses to the prospect of death and death itself differ within and between societies. Reduced infant mortality rates (IMRs) and increasing longevity in the western world over the past 150 years, largely the result of improvements in the general quality of life, hygiene and sanitation, have changed the way in which we experience death. The availability of new health technologies in end-of-life care has profound implications for individuals, families and carers, while social and behavioural factors affect the use of these technologies.

Lecture Notes: The Social Basis of Medicine, 1st edition. By Andrew Russell. Published 2009 by Blackwell Publishing. ISBN: 978-1-4051-3912-0

This chapter covers the following topics

The changing experience of death in the UK and elsewhere
Likely psychological responses to the threat of fatal illness
Bereavement, grief and mourning
In search of the 'good' death

The changing experience of death in the UK and elsewhere

Changing mortality rates in the UK, 1841 compared to 2001

1841: 22 deaths per 1000 population, nearly one half of these from infectious diseases.
2001: 12 deaths per 1000 population, with death from infectious diseases very rare.

In the early Victorian period, the likelihood of witnessing others dying during one's lifetime was much higher than it is in the UK today. While there were considerable differences between the classes, the chance of at least one of your children dying before you did was high. Maternal mortality (death in childbirth) was also a real possibility. Today, the death of a child is a much rarer and in many ways more tragic event, while the death of a mother in childbirth is extremely unusual and is commonly regarded as a failure on the part of the medical profession.

Across the world, longevity has increased from an average of 48 years in 1955 to 65 years in 1995. However, Table 13.1 shows there is still considerable variation between Europe and Africa in terms of life expectancy and age structures. Much of this is due to differences in infant mortality rate (IMR). A child born in Africa is nearly eight times more likely to die before reaching its first birthday than a child born in Europe. For this reason, the overall life expectancy at birth is nearly 20 years less in Africa than in Europe, and is falling further in many countries due to HIV/AIDS. Because of the likelihood of a child dying young, as well as for other economic and cultural reasons, fertility rates among African women are higher than among European women and hence the proportion of children in African countries is greater than in Europe. The proportion of elderly people is correspondingly much lower.

Of course, such generalizations mask considerable differences. The Republic of South Africa, for example, is closer to a European demographic profile, whereas 16 countries experienced a decline in their life expectancy between 1975 and 1995, many of these in Eastern Europe and Russia. There is also considerable variation within countries, as South Africa also demonstrates.

It is not only in numerical terms that death has changed in the UK since the nineteenth century; how we die has also changed. In its increasing confinement to old age, death is now more likely to follow a lengthy illness, one that may involve considerable suffering and dependency (see Chapter 12) – a shift from a 'quick death' to a 'slow death' (Table 13.2). People are far more likely to die in hospital or a hospice, and hence death may be said to have gone from being 'visible' to 'invisible'. Finally, death itself has come to be defined differently and more problematically. The development of medical technology has had a part to play in this change.

In 2000, two-thirds of deaths in the UK occurred in hospital. The proportion of hospice deaths, while increasing slowly, is still relatively low. Most people express the hope that they will die in their own home, yet less than one-fifth manage

Table 13.1 Some key demographic statistics: Europe and Africa compared (Source: WHO 1998, World Health Statistics).

	Distribution (%) of age group 0–14	Distribution (%) of age group 15–64	Distribution (%) of age group 65+	Life expectancy (years) at birth (1995–2000)	IMR per 1000 births (1995–2000)
Africa	43.7	53.2	3.2	53.8	85.6
Europe	18.9	67.1	14.0	72.6	11.6

Table 13.2 From 'quick death' to 'slow death'.

Quick death associated with	Slow death associated with
Pre-modern era	Modern era
Low levels of medical technology	High levels of medical technology
Late detection of disease	Early detection of disease
Simple definition of death (e.g. cessation of heart beat)	Complex definitions of death
High levels of acute disease mortality	High levels of chronic disease mortality
High incidence of fatal injuries	Low incidence of fatal injuries
Relative passivity towards a person once in the 'dying' category, or their killing or suicide	Activist, curative orientation towards person in the 'dying' category with high value put on prolongation of life

Source: Adapted from Lofland (1978)

Table 13.3 Changing place of death: UK, 1990–2000.

Place of Death	1990 (All deaths %)	2000 (All deaths %)
Hospital	54	66.5
Hospice	4	4.3
Other communal establishments	14	7.8
Home	23	19.0
Other private houses	5	2.4

Source: National Statistics website: www.statistics.gov.uk.

to do so and the proportion is declining. Despite the trend towards 'slow death' (see Table 13.2), Table 13.3 reminds us that, at the same time, death has become increasingly 'invisible' as it has shifted from community settings to institutions. The 'can do' culture of medicine has a part to play here. Death, particularly the death of a child, is increasingly regarded as something that should be preventable. The development of cryogenics, which allows seriously ill patients to pay to have their bodies deep frozen until the day when a cure can be found for their malady, is a symptom of this trend. (As this is an exorbitantly expensive procedure, it is confined to the very wealthy.) Hospitals are a wonderful institutional means for the rest of society to act as if death did not exist. Within hospitals the dying are frequently removed from public view into side-rooms where they can die, ideally surrounded by grieving relatives, who thus avoid embarrassing public demonstrations of emotion. While religion remains a comfort to some, the increasing secularization of society means that for many the 'Why me?' 'Why him or her?' 'Why now?' questions have become far more difficult to answer.

Changing definitions of death: the role of health technologies

Prior to the nineteenth century, death was regarded as a biological process (putrefaction) rather than a time-specific event. The introduction of the stethoscope offered a specific point of death – the cessation of the heart beat. With the

development of ventilators and other forms of life-support machinery in the twentieth century the concept of 'brain death' has been invented, although the criteria for determining brain death differ between nations and only about 1% of deaths in the UK are ever defined in this way. Were it not for the 'persistent vegetative state' (which life-support technology permits) and the rise in techniques of organ transplantation, it is doubtful whether 'brain death' would exist at all. Some intensive care physicians regard death as a two-stage process – brain death, an irreversible diagnosis where the 'person' no longer exists, and cardiopulmonary death, when the body dies. The anomalous status of the organ donor as both 'living' and 'dead' is problematic for family and health professionals alike.

Medical technology is not the only factor determining how death is defined, however. In the UK, consensus is that biological death has occurred when there is irreversible cessation of higher brain activity. Although the medical technologies are similar, in the US whole brain death is regarded as the determining factor. In Shinto Japan, death is regarded as a natural process of conversion into an ancestor. The soul/mind (*reikon*) exists throughout the entire body, and only leaves when the corpse is cold and stiffening. Reincarnation requires a favourable state of consciousness to be carried into the next life. If a person does not die intact, they will not pass into the next life. If part of the body is still alive in someone else, then the donor is not fully dead. For these reasons, transplant surgery is virtually unknown in Japan.

The development of technology to support life in situations where people might previously have died raises difficult ethical decisions, such as when to withdraw or stop treatment, the status of 'do not resuscitate' orders, euthanasia, and the like. The ethics of end-of-life issues is becoming a speciality in its own right (see *Lecture Notes: Medical Law and Ethics*, Chapters 11 and 12).

Social death

Death may also be defined in social rather than biological terms. Social death is the elimination of the social existence of a person in other people's lives and may occur well before biological death. Social death has as much to do with how the person is treated by others (exclusion) as it does with the actions of the person themselves. Thus retirement, death of a spouse, imprisonment or entry into a retirement home are all examples of varying degrees of social death in the UK. Diagnosis of an incurable disease such as incipient dementia may also affect the way people treat the person and thus expedite their social death. The nocebo effect (the reverse of the positive, placebo affect – see Chapter 5), which occurs when patients believe things are going to get worse, may seriously deplete the health of the individual. Curses, like negative prognoses, may play their part in hastening a person's demise. In Aboriginal Australia, for example, a person accused of wrongdoing may be condemned and quite literally be 'sung' to death. In the Scottish Hebrides, until recently, access to medical services was such that the air ambulance was summoned only as a last resort. To be taken away in the ambulance plane was regarded by many elderly people as tantamount to being taken away to die.

Social death also occurs with admission in hospital. The shift from person to patient is inherently a reduction in that person's social repertoire. The social existence of dying patients in particular is often reduced or eliminated owing to the frequently subtle ways in which other parties withdraw from them physically, emotionally and communicatively. As we have seen above, the procedure in many hospitals has been to transfer dying patients from the main ward to a side-room, and for health care professionals to withdraw from the patient and family. This is the point at which the hospice model of 'intensive palliative care' should come into force, with its aim of providing care that enlarges rather than reduces the social existence of the terminally ill patient and his or her relatives, while addressing their physical, psychological and spiritual needs. However, social death prior to physical death remains the norm rather than the exception.

Social death may also occur well after biological death, however. Examples include bereaved parents, spouses or children maintaining a relationship of sorts with dead relatives – talking to them, attending their grave and doing things in their memory. In some religions, such as Shinto-ism (see above), social death may never occur if the person is regarded as having become an ancestor or where there is a belief in reincarnation. In 'last offices', the standardized procedures for dealing with the dead in a clinical context, the body is laid out, washed and tidied, straightened and protected. It is made safe for others to handle and for others to see. The environment the body is in is made as calm and pleasant as possible. Nurses have been observed talking to the body while undertaking last offices. Indeed, having regard for the corpse as a 'dead person' rather than just a 'dead body' is of great importance. Part of the distress felt by relatives of babies and young children who had body parts removed after death at Alder Hey hospital without the parents' consent was the disregard for this principle. Clearly, for most people who die, elements of a social existence are maintained after biological death has taken place.

Likely psychological responses to the threat of fatal illness

Every patient is different in their response to the threat of fatal illness, but certain patterns can be discerned. Two things need to be considered in understanding the responses patients may make. The first is the degree of awareness they have that they are dying; the second is the personal, social and cultural context in which they face the prospect of death.

Awareness of dying

Types of awareness

- Closed awareness
- Suspected awareness
- Mutual pretence awareness
- Open awareness

The types of awareness of dying are only partly related to the communication skills of the doctor or other carers. Uncertainty affords hope to the patient. In Japan, patients who are terminally ill with cancer are traditionally *not* told they are dying, because of the strong belief among both health professionals and the lay public that hopelessness leads to premature death. There is evidence from around the world that death comes more quickly to those who 'give up' on life. Different forms of death awareness have been identified that influence this process. 'Closed awareness' is where the patient is unaware that they are dying, but their carers know. This knowledge may lead to carers treating the dying patient differently from how they treat a patient they do not believe to be dying. 'Suspected awareness', as the term suggests, is when the patient suspects they are dying but is uncertain (and hence may continue to hope they are not). In situations of 'mutual pretence awareness', both patient and carers know the patient is dying but pretend they aren't. In 'open awareness' both patient and others are aware the patient is dying. Even within open awareness, however, shock may lead to a suspension of knowledge. Such patients, though they know they are dying, may remain in denial. Doubts may arise and the patient reverts to a different form of awareness when there is an unexpected improvement or deterioration in their condition. Such suspended open awareness may be the permanently preferred option, with reality being called into question. Active open awareness involves abandonment of all hope of improvement.

Personal, social and cultural context of dying

Factors affecting individual responses to the threat of fatal illness

- Physical and mental symptoms and consequent distress
- Age
- Family intimacy and support
- Religious convictions
- The 'stage of dying' the individual has reached

Table 13.4 Symptoms experienced in the last year of life in the UK (1990).

	Cancer %	Heart disease %	Stroke %
Pain	88	77	66
Breathlessness	54	60	37
Nausea/vomiting	59	32	23
Difficulty swallowing	41	16	23
Constipation	63	38	45
Mental confusion	41	32	50
Pressure sores	28	11	20
Urinary incontinence	40	30	56
Bowel incontinence	32	17	37

Source: Addington-Hall (1996)

Table 13.4 is based on a retrospective study of nearly 3000 people conducted in 1990. What is apparent is that symptoms experienced by people suffering different end-of-life diseases vary tremendously. The 'symptom load' is generally greater for cancer sufferers than for those with heart disease or stroke, except that those with heart disease are more likely to experience breathlessness as a result of their illness, while those with stroke are more likely to experience mental confusion and incontinence. These differences may help to explain the greater fear of cancer than of heart disease among the lay public in the UK even though, in 2000, marginally more people died of heart disease (26 per cent of deaths) than died of cancer (25 per cent). Certainly the symptoms, and the way they are dealt with by the medical profession and other carers, will affect the experience of dying from these illnesses among individual patients.

Age

Children with life-limiting diseases such as muscular dystrophy and cystic fibrosis are faced with death at a young age. Their age and cognitive state affects their likely reaction to this. 'Death' is a very abstract concept and as such tends not to be well understood by very young children. Only by about eight years of age does the child understand that everyone dies, that death is final (i.e. not a temporary visit to somewhere else) and involves the absence of bodily functions. While some children will have had some experience of death (e.g. the death of a grandparent, neighbour or a pet), they will not always have been fully appraised of what has happened. They may have been told the dead person has 'gone away' or is 'sleeping for a long time'. Even though they may not be told they have a terminal illness, dying school-age children generally seem to understand the serious nature of their illness and to be far more anxious than seriously ill children who are not dying. The development of the children's hospice movement attests to their special needs.

The five stages of dying

- Denial and isolation
- Anger
- Bargaining
- Depression
- Acceptance

The five stages of dying were identified by Elisabeth Kübler-Ross, who conducted a major study of terminally ill adults and their carers. The first stage, denial and isolation, commonly occurs on first hearing the news that one is terminally ill. It corresponds to the state of suspended open awareness (discussed above), and persisted to the very end in 3 out of the 200 patients in Kübler-Ross's study. Anger occurs at the second stage and stems from the 'Why me?' question. Much of the brunt of this anger is borne by the patient's carers. Anger leads into the bargaining stage: possible examples include setting up (sometimes secret) pacts with God, and offering to donate one's body to science on the expectation of even more diligent care from health workers. Depression is the understandable development of a sense of loss and anticipatory grief. There may also be reactive depression to surgery or physical or mental weakness. Acceptance is a sort of peace. Hopefully, the pain is fully under control and the struggle is over. It is a stage marked by weakness and a diminished interest in the world. At this stage, the family often needs support more than the patient.

The 'stages of dying' model has been influential. However, people do not follow these stages in a consistent way. Some may not follow the implied chronology at all or may exhibit aspects of several of the stages at the same time. Patients may move back and forth through the stages, reverting to denial if they think they are getting better.

Case Study: Jean

Jean is dying of lung cancer. She has a daughter, Trudi, aged nine, whom she has chosen not to tell about her impending death. Jean has been with her partner, who is not Trudi's biological father, for eight years.

Trudi's biological father is in prison. What happens to the daughter after her death? Unless she is legally adopted by the partner who loves her as a father, legally she 'belongs' to the biological father. What if he isn't a fit person? Does the child have any say? If so, who should be involved in these discussions?

What might be some of the different answers to Jean's questions?

Bereavement, grief and mourning

The stages of dying model has also been applied to the grieving process. Death to the patient is bereavement to his or her loved ones. Health professionals may also be affected by the death of a patient. Grief is the psychological response to bereavement, and may follow Kübler-Ross's model quite closely. Mourning is the public expression of bereavement. As such, it is subject to customs and norms just like other forms of social activity, and varies both cross-culturally and historically.

Factors affecting the grieving process

- Nature of relationship – duration, depth and quality
- Circumstances of death
- Personality and background
- Life after bereavement

The nature of the relationship

The closer the relationship, the more grief there is likely to be. The closeness of the relationship is not necessarily linked to its duration. A stillbirth or perinatal death will have a devastating affect on the parents, who will be grieving a wholly unfulfilled future. Where the relationship with a dead person was difficult when they were alive, the loss of potential for the relationship ever to be repaired may be another dimension to the grief experienced.

Circumstances of death

The circumstances of the death can be looked at in a variety of ways. If someone has experienced a slow death, some stages of the Kübler-Ross model may already have been traversed and the grieving may appear less acute than if the death is quick or unexpected (e.g. following an accident). Sometimes death results in financial hardship or housing problems for those who remain. Where legal complications are present, such as the need for an inquest, compensation claims or litigation, these may add to the stress the family experiences. Suicide, and the taboo that often accompanies it, is a particularly traumatic cause of bereavement and one that may be very difficult for family and friends to come to terms with. Anger is also a significant emotion in cases of bereavement by suicide.

Personality and background

How a person learned to deal with loss in childhood will affect how they deal with grief in adulthood. Culture and beliefs about death also determine how we grieve. Physical and mental health play a part, as do previous experiences of grief and any unresolved loss.

Life after bereavement

Finally, the prospects for the person following the bereavement, the social networks that they can draw on and the directions their life is likely to take will impact on the nature and extent of the grieving process.

In search of the 'good' death

In recent years attention has shifted from the significance of quick or slow death to the notion of a 'good death'. This is something that not only patients but also their families, physicians and other carers will have strong views about. Providing an environment where the experience of death is as good as possible for the dying patient and those they leave behind is a key way in which health professionals can play a positive role. If there is a sense that the death was 'good', then the grieving process is likely to be mitigated. A number of factors have been identified that are likely to lead to a good death. However, ideas about the 'good death' are heavily dependent on society and culture, and for members of some minority groups the prospect of experiencing a 'good death' is limited.

What makes a good death?

- Control of symptoms
- Preparation for death
- Opportunity for closure or 'sense of completion' of a life well-lived
- Good relationship with health care professionals

Culture and the good death

What is classified as a 'good' or 'bad' death is highly dependent on religious beliefs and ideas of personal autonomy. Only about 40% of those living in Europe believe in an afterlife or any form of reincarnation. Religion is increasingly a personal choice, and in the UK health care chaplaincies and the hospice movement work to help patients discover their own spirituality and path through illness and death. There is increasing emphasis on the personal autonomy of the dying – a key element to a 'good death' is being in control, and a patient who lacks autonomy, because of stroke or Alzheimer's disease, say, experiences a 'bad' death.

The good death in minority cultures

Western societies are increasingly multicultural, and notions of what constitutes a good death for the majority may not be shared by members of minority groups such as Hindus or Muslims. There is a danger of 'cultural stereotyping' of the sort that says 'all Hindus believe x' or 'all Muslims do y'. There are many different types of Hinduism, as there are all world religions. Yet it is important to try to understand some of ways in which religious beliefs and practices among minority groups may influence the possibility of experiencing a 'good' death.

Case study: The good death in Hindu communities

- Preferably in Varanasi (Benares), India, or with access to water from the Ganges
- Death should be freely given ('relinquish the body')
- Preferably on the floor
- Dying outside, or at home, preferred to death in hospital
- On death, religious state is important – should hear the name of God chanted by family members
- Death rituals managed by family, not funeral directors
- Glass-topped coffin preferred
- Death occurs when the soul (*pran*) leaves the body, ideally during the *kapal kriya* (breaking of the skull ritual, halfway through cremation)

How might these differences be taken into account in UK health care settings?

The clinical responsibilities and dilemmas in managing a 'good' death

Death in the UK is an increasingly medicalized experience. GPs may find themselves attending up to five deaths a year. Their hospital colleagues are likely to attend many more. Even doctors who have little contact with death in their clinical practice may be asked to give an 'expert' statement for the coroner service. Death thus affects all doctors, to varying degrees. It also affects them emotionally, irrespective of their seniority, although junior doctors and senior attending physicians differ in how much social support they need and use. Female doctors experience more psychological distress than their male counterparts, irrespective of seniority, and report needing and receiving more support, particularly from their colleagues. For the doctor, the length of time

spent taking care of a dying patient is associated with greater satisfaction with the end-of-life care provided and increased likelihood of experiencing the death as an emotional loss, with linked symptoms of grief and trauma. There is a 'conspiracy of silence' towards emotions in medicine which can cause unnecessary stress, maladaptive coping strategies and burnout from the cumulative effects of emotionally draining deaths. Good practice indicates the benefit of medical teams debriefing within their department in order to give all staff involved the opportunity to share their responses and reflections on the patient's death.

Apart from its impact on medical personnel themselves, death is an area in which the interaction of medicine and society is at its strongest and most blatant. If health professionals are to respond sensitively to this most difficult period in people's lives, it is necessary to consider both what the medicalization of death entails and how the socialization of medicine can maximize the chances of facilitating a 'good death' in every case.

The social functions of medicine in death and dying

Initial assessment and care

The two key questions patients and their families have of the medical profession are 'Am I dying?' and 'How long have I got?' The diagnosis of dying is a vital first step in the shift of management goals from 'cure' to 'palliative care'. It is dependent on the recognition of key signs and symptoms according to the nature of the chronic incurable disease from which the patient is suffering, and is a clinical skill that may take years to develop. Death from cancer, for example, is usually the result of a gradual deterioration of function (see below).

Signs associated with dying phase of cancer patients

- Patient becomes bed-bound
- Patient is semi-comatose
- Patient is able to take sips of fluid only
- Patient is no longer able to take drugs orally

Some cancer patients die suddenly (e.g. because of a massive haemorrhage), and death and dying from all conditions is subject to the vagaries of the individual patient who does not fit the 'norm'. Heart disease is an example of a condition where the diagnosis of dying is more complex and often problematic. The palliative care needs of patients with heart failure have until recently been neglected despite this being the most common cause of death in many secondary care wards. In many cases, worsening heart failure may be due to a proximate cause that is reversible and may lead to symptomatic remission.

Examples of reasons for reversible causes of worsening heart failure

Chest infection
Anaemia
Arrhythmia
Suboptimal drugs
Inappropriate drugs or use of drugs

In addition, standard diuretics, inotropes and vasodilators may produce a temporary improvement in the patient's condition.

With experience, clinicians in secondary care may come to recognize a subgroup of heart failure patients with a particularly poor prognosis.

Characteristics of heart failure patients with poor prognosis

Previous admissions to hospital with worsening heart failure
No identifiable reversible precipitant
Receiving optimum tolerated conventional drugs
Deteriorating renal function
Failure to respond within two or three days to appropriate changes in diuretic or vasodilator

---

There are numerous other ways in which the initial assessment and care of dying patients may be inhibited, due to the culture of medicine. The focus on 'cure' in medical practice (see Chapter 4)

may lead to the pursuit of unrealistic or futile interventions in the hope that the patient will get better. Health care professionals may be reluctant to diagnose dying because they are inadequately trained in palliative care techniques and therefore feel helpless. Lack of a definitive diagnosis or disagreements about the patient's condition within the multidisciplinary team may also inhibit the diagnosis of dying, leading to 'mixed messages' being communicated to patients and their families, and poor management practices due to opposed goals of care.

Where the prospects for recovery are uncertain, it is better to discuss this rather than offering false hope to a patient and his or her family. For example, in the case of heart disease patients exhibiting one or more of the poor prognosis characteristics indicated above, clinicians should review and discuss with patients and carers the chances of recovery and hence the justification for continuing invasive treatments or monitoring. Whatever the condition, poor communication skills may prevent the doctor from articulating a diagnosis of dying and discussing the options with patients and carers. This leads to the ultimate weakening of trust in the doctor–patient relationship, an increased risk that the patient will die an undignified death with uncontrolled symptoms and the overall prospect of a 'bad' death.

In response to the question 'How long have I got?' the doctor has another difficult clinical task to perform: predicting survival in the terminally ill. Accurately predicting when death will occur is important for good clinical decision-making. Evidence suggests that doctors' survival predictions for patients with terminal cancer tend to be inaccurate, often overestimating the survival time, although they become more accurate as death approaches. Inaccuracy in this regard is another way in which prospects for a 'good death' may be impaired.

Ongoing care of the dying patient

The intensive palliative care model provides for the physical, psychological, social and spiritual care of patients and their relatives. Some patients may have written an advance care statement. These can be useful in facilitating discussions about care. However, they are based on assumptions within medical culture about autonomy and individual decision-making, which may be problematic. Older people in a Sheffield study, for example, expressed reservations about the completion of such statements. They could see their potential for supporting personal integrity and in helping families reduce the burden of decision-making when death approached. On the other hand, thinking about, let alone discussing, death and dying was difficult for them. They were concerned about whether clinical actions following adherence to an advance care statement might be akin to euthanasia. Furthermore, they were worried that their preferences might change as death approached. The study concluded that a processual approach to advance care planning, involving clinicians, patients and families in ongoing discussion and review, is preferable to the creation of a 'once and for all' advance statement.

The following list provides a satisfactory biopsychosocial approach to dying and death that is appropriate for all settings. Particular requirements for community settings are indented.

Physical care

- Current medication assessed and non-essential drugs discontinued.
- Oral medications (e.g. opioids, anxiolytics and antiemetics) converted to a subcutaneous route, and a syringe driver employed for continuous infusion if appropriate.
- Inappropriate interventions (e.g. blood tests, antibiotics, intravenous fluids and drugs, turning regimens, measurement of vital signs) discontinued.
- Document patient 'not for cardiopulmonary resuscitation'.
- Inform the GP of the patient's condition:
  ○ ensure 'as required' drugs are readily available in the patient's home;
  ○ make a round-the-clock district nursing services available;
  ○ ensure continuity of care within GP out-of-hours services.

Psychological care

- Ensure communication is adequate (e.g. is a translator needed?).
- Assess patient's and family's insight into the patient's condition and explore issues concerning dying and death sensitively and appropriately.

Social care

- Discuss with the family the clinical expectation that their loved one is dying and will die.
- Avoid use of ambiguous language (e.g. 'may not get better') which can lead to misinterpretation and confusion:
  ○ Give relatives contact telephone numbers so that they have access to help and advice round the clock.

Spiritual care

- Discuss religious and spiritual needs with patient and their family, with sensitivity to the patient's cultural and religious background.
  ○ Are there any formal religious practices appropriate for the dying phase or that may influence care of the body after death?

Care after death

After death, care shifts to the bereaved, who should be cared for in a compassionate manner. Literature about issues relating to grieving may be helpful. However, the clinician also has to deal with death as a medical and statutory matter. This may involve post-mortem examination, issuing a medical certificate, completing cremation forms, notifying and writing a report for the coroner, and an inquest (12% of reported deaths in the UK require an inquest – see below). In addition to custody issues involving surviving children (see Case study: Jean, above), the bereaved relatives usually have other legal issues to deal with, such as wills, the reassessment of benefits allowances, insurance claims, etc. The increasing number of unmarried partners of the opposite sex and same-sex couples may have particular problems in this area in a legal system that generally caters for married couples rather than unmarried partners.

The death of a child poses particular strains on families and medical staff alike. It is also important that where children have been bereaved, their needs and concerns are taken into account in dealing with the death.

Issuing a medical certificate of cause of death

All doctors who have been in attendance at the last illness of a patient have a statutory duty to issue a medical certificate of cause of death (MCCD) for the Registrar of Births, Marriages and Deaths. The MCCD gives the cause of death to the best of the doctor's knowledge. Sometimes the MCCD will contain medical terms that relatives do not understand. It is therefore important to translate the contents of the MCCD to the relatives in everyday language. Assessing the cause of death has become a much more exact science, and ambiguous or vague phrases such as 'old age' or 'frailty' are no longer acceptable, although these may be found on the medical certificates of the past. An MCCD requires the doctor to:

- Have made a diagnosis prior to death.
- Be satisfied that no other condition or event contributed significantly to the death that is not a natural disease.
- Have expected the death to occur at roughly the time it did.
- Be satisfied that the mode and circumstances of death are compatible with the diagnosis.

The coroner

If the doctor is unable to certify the cause of death for one or more of the above reasons, he or she should refer the case to the coroner. Every borough in England has an assigned coroner (in Scotland, this role is occupied by the procurator fiscal). The coroner is a registered lawyer and may also be a doctor. The coroner's job it is to establish the medical cause of death if it is unknown or if the death was 'unnatural'. The following are occasions when the coroner should be notified:

- When the certifying doctor has not seen the patient professionally in the 14 days leading up to death.
- Where the cause of death remains unknown.
- If the death occurred after surgery.
- When the cause of death may have been unnatural or suspicious.
- Where the death may have occurred from industrial disease or poisoning.

If a death is reported to the coroner, the Registrar is unable to complete his or her work until after the coroner's inquiry. This may take some time, and it is important that relatives are put in touch with the coroner as soon as possible, after which funeral arrangements, including a likely date, can be discussed in order to reduce the amount of unnecessary distress the bereaved experience. The coroner may ask a pathologist to perform a post-mortem examination. If this shows that the death was due to natural causes, an MCCD will be issued. Burial or cremation can then take place. If the post-mortem shows any cause for suspicion, then an inquiry will be ordered, although the coroner will probably allow the body to be buried or cremated if there is no indication of a need for further examinations.

The inquest

The aim of an inquest is to uncover the information required by the Registrar of Deaths so that a death can be formally registered. It is a fact-finding inquiry, not a judicial proceeding, that seeks answers to questions with regard to the death ('Who?' 'Where?' 'When?' and 'How?'). The coroner will usually sit alone, although under certain circumstances a jury will be formed to decide the final verdict.

Juries are required in the following circumstances:

- Death resulting from an incident at work.
- Death occurring while in custody.
- Death occurring on a railway.
- Any other death that has associated circumstances that could be detrimental to the health and safety of the public.

All 'properly interested persons' may be called as witnesses to an inquiry, including life insurance issuers and claimants and those whose actions may have contributed to the death. Inquiries are normally held in public and the press may be present. The aim of the inquest is to uncover the information required by the Registrar, so that the death can be formally registered.

Cremation forms

About 70% of deaths in the UK today are followed by a cremation. Every cremation legally requires a cremation certificate issued by a medical referee. The medical referee works for the local cremation authority and must have been a registered medical practitioner for at least five years. For the referee to issue a certificate, the death certificate and a completed cremation form are required, following which the medical referee must be satisfied that the cause of death is as stated. The first part of the cremation form is normally completed by the doctor responsible for the MCCD. The second part has to be completed by a second doctor, who must also have been registered at least five years. This doctor must discuss the circumstances of death with the first doctor, examine the body and sign the certificate to confirm he or she agrees with the cause of death. The coroner is the point of contact for advice if there are any doubts about whether or not the cause of death can be certified.

Case study: A bad death in a Muslim community

'On Saturday a young Pakistani friend of ours died unexpectedly. She had arrived from Pakistan two years ago with her two young sons. She was in hospital for eight weeks and it was believed that she had a "blood disorder". Unfortunately, things were serious and she died. When my family went on Saturday they said the family were in a lot of distress as the hospital would not allow the corpse to be released without a post-mortem. The family were in dispute with the hospital and local community leaders had to attend. The funeral could not take place until Monday, which was deemed to be 'painful' for the corpse. According to Islam the funeral should preferably take place as soon as possible, and at the funeral her family and others were saying that a post-mortem should not have taken place, especially (also for religious reasons) because the body was that of a woman. This was an extremely upsetting time for the local British Pakistani community.'

How could the hospital have handled this case in a more culturally sensitive manner?

Summary

- Medicine impacts on society in terms of the nature, definition and experience of death today. The medicalization of death requires a sensitive evaluation of what this means for patients, relatives and health professionals.

- Social norms and values permeate the practice of medicine in situations of death and dying. Doctors are responsible for dealing with death not only at the individual or family level, but also as a statutory process.

- Psychological processes can be identified that help to explain different responses to the stages of dying and to bereavement, grief and mourning.

- The 'good' death, notions of which vary within and between cultures, should be an aspirational goal of all health care professionals.

Further reading

Addington-Hall, J. (1996) Heart disease and stroke: lessons from cancer care. In G. Ford and I. Lewin (eds) *Managing Terminal Illness*. London: Royal College of Physicians.

Ariès, P. (1983) *The Hour of Our Death*. Harmondsworth: Penguin Books.

British Medical Journal (2003) Special issue: What is a good death? *British Medical Journal*, **327(7408)**.

Buckman, R. (1984) Breaking bad news: why is it still so difficult? *British Medical Journal*, **288(1)**: 172–9.

Charlton, R. and Smith, G. (2002) Dealing with deaths. *BMJ Career Focus*, **325**:107.

Child Bereavement Charity http://www.childbereavement.org.uk. Accessed 27 November 2007.

Dickenson, D., Johnson, M. and Katz, J. S. (2000) *Death, Dying and Bereavement* (2nd edn.). London: Open University Press in association with Sage.

Ellershaw, J. and Ward, C. (2003) Care of the dying patient: the last hours or days of life. *British Medical Journal*, **326**: 30–4.

Helman, C. (2001) *Culture, Health and Illness* (4th edn.). London: Arnold, pp. 161–4.

Henley, A. and Schott, J. (1999) *Culture, Religion and Patient Care in a Multi-Ethnic Society: a Handbook for Professionals*. London: Age Concern Books, Chapter 18: Care for people who are dying.

Howard, P. and Bogle, J. (2004) *Lecture Notes: Medical Law and Ethics*. Oxford: Blackwell.

Kübler-Ross, E. (1997) *On Death and Dying – What the Dying Have to Teach Doctors, Nurses, Clergy, and Their Own Families*. New York: Scribner Classics.

Lock, M. (2002) Inventing a new death and making it believable. *Anthropology and Medicine*, **9(2)**: 97–115.

Lofland, L. (1978) *The Craft of Dying: the Modern Face of Death*. Beverly Hills, CA: Sage.

Mulkay, M. (1993) Social death in Britain. In D. Clark (ed.) *The Sociology of Death*. Oxford: Blackwell.

Neuberger, J. (1987) *Caring for Dying People of Different Faiths*. London: Lisa Sainsbury Foundation.

Scambler, G. (2003) Dying, death and bereavement. In G. Scambler (ed.) *Sociology as Applied to Medicine* (5th edn). London: Saunders.

Seale, C. (2000) Changing patterns of death and dying. *Social Science and Medicine*, **51**: 917–30.

Seymour, J., Gott, M., Bellamy, G., Ahmedzai, S. H. and Clark, D. (2004) Planning for the end of life: the views of older people about advance care statements. *Social Science and Medicine*, **59**: 57–68.

Chapter 14

International health

Introduction

The contemporary world is marked by the compression of space and time. This phenomenon is known as globalization, a process associated with the greater and increasingly rapid movement of people, objects and ideas, both within and between countries around the world. This process has been facilitated by various technological revolutions over the past 500 years or so which have led to transport, communications and media developments spanning the globe. Whereas in the past it might have taken six months to travel from England to Australia by sailing ship, a journey which few would have been likely to accomplish in their lifetime, today it is a journey that can be made in 24 hours by jumbo jet.

People have traditionally associated travel with illness. During the colonial period, for example, West Africa was colloquially known as the 'white man's grave'. Much of the knowledge of tropical illnesses today stems from research and practice originally carried out in the name of colonial medical services established to serve the needs of British colonies around the world. However, the problems faced by the British colonialists were as nothing compared to the devastating epidemics wrought by 'western' diseases such as measles and

smallpox on immunologically naïve indigenous populations during European exploration and expansion between 1500 and 1800. In the other direction, syphilis was a disease previously unknown in the West but endemic in Central and South America which was spread globally by returning seafarers. Today, immunological naivety is as much a feature of many of the inhabitants of richer countries as it is of the tiny number of indigenous populations that remain largely untouched by the global economy. Thirty-two new diseases have been identified since 1970 (approximately one a year), including potentially fatal ones such as severe acute respiratory syndrome (SARS) and HIV/AIDS. Their aetiology and distribution make them all potentially international as well as lower-level health problems, especially given the increasing interconnectedness and movement of people around the world today.

The increasing mobility of people, allied with burgeoning human populations, is reflected in greater degrees of urbanization and the increasing social and cultural diversity of people living in urban areas. In recent decades the economics of one group of the most heavily populated developing countries have grown than those of developed countries. Other poor countries are being left behind economically, however, and within countries there are increasing disparities too: many people in rural areas are lagging behind their urban counterparts, for example.

Lecture Notes: The Social Basis of Medicine, 1st edition. By Andrew Russell. Published 2009 by Blackwell Publishing. ISBN: 978-1-4051-3912-0

The effects of globalization on health are complex and contested. There have been some spectacular success stories, from concerted efforts to eradicate specific infectious diseases – the last recorded case of smallpox occurred in 1977 and polio is nearly eradicated. However, the gains from global economic growth have been highly unequally distributed, and while there have been significant improvements in global health overall, including life expectancy, some countries have seen a sharp drop in such indicators, often as a result of HIV/AIDS and the resurgence of associated infectious diseases such as tuberculosis. The growing disparities between rich and poor, both within and between countries, have serious implications for health and well-being (see Chapter 7). Furthermore, in the long term the poorest countries are those most likely to be vulnerable to the effects of climate change (which is fuelled by the economic development experienced by others) and least able to offset its effects.

The increasing flow of knowledge and levels of movement have led to a growing interest among medical students about issues affecting health and health care across the world as well as in their own countries. Many take electives and professional 'gap years' overseas in order to gain experience and leadership credentials in the field. The International Federation of Medical Students' Associations is a federation of student-led organizations involved in debate and action on global health.

This chapter covers the following topics

Globalization and its effects on health and health care in rich countries

Globalization and its effects on health and health care in poor countries

---

Globalization and its effects on health and health care in rich countries

Travel medicine

The popularity of international travel continues to grow. In 2006, there were 846 million 'international arrivals' (movements across frontiers recorded by authorities), representing a 6.5% growth rate year on year for over 50 years. Assuming this trend continues, the figure will have doubled again by 2020. However, such journeying is still very much an elite activity. In 1996, only 3.5% of the world's total population travelled abroad, 80% of them from 17 European nations, the US, Canada or Japan. In 2005, UK citizens made 66 million trips overseas – more than one trip for every person in the country. The travelling population is also changing, with increasing numbers of elderly and immuno-compromised people seeking exotic holidays and increasing the demand for specialized travel medicine services.

As people visit more exotic and remote parts of the world doctors need to understand the diseases of travel both to be able to serve the needs of individual patients and as a public health issue. Exposure among travellers to diseases that are rare in the developed world is rising, especially where the traveller's behaviour or special epidemiological characteristics of the country visited play a part. Furthermore, travellers can introduce these diseases into their community on their return, thus posing a potential public health threat.

Travel to less developed countries and health

Data from the 1980s and 1990s indicate that, for every 100,000 travellers from developed countries spending a month visiting less developed countries:

- 50,000 will have a health problem during their visit
- 8000 will seek medical care
- 5000 will be bedridden
- 1100 will be incapacitated in their work either abroad or on return
- 300 will be admitted to hospital during the trip or on return
- 50 will have to be air evacuated
- 1 will die.

While many infectious diseases are now considered 'vaccine-preventable', there is a tendency for some travellers to demand vaccines for every disease found in the country or countries they are visiting whether or not they are likely to come into contact with them. For example, while the prevalence of meningococcal infection in East Africa is high, its incidence among tourists is virtually zero, but many will insist on 'jabs' for this and other rare diseases. Others meanwhile ignore the risks and potential for prevention of all sorts, or need to travel at short notice which poses its own problems, although it is now possible to provide good levels of protection within four weeks. However, travel medicine is about more than the prevention of travel-related infections, since there are many other potential hazards that travellers may encounter. A ritual series of vaccinations does not absolve travellers from the need to behave safely once they have arrived in what may be an unfamiliar environment, and health education of various sorts is often necessary.

Malaria: a concern for international health

Malaria is a disease predominantly affecting people living in or visiting Africa, South and Central America, Asia and the Middle East. The heaviest burden is in Africa, where around 90% of the approximately one million deaths from malaria worldwide occur each year, due largely to the effects of *falciparum* malaria, which is capable of invading a high proportion of red blood cells and rapidly leading to severe or life-threatening multi-organ disease. Exact numbers are hard to establish, but latest research estimates that 2.2 billion people, most of them living in developing countries, are at risk. In 2002, there were over 500 million cases of *Plasmodium falciparum* malaria globally, two-thirds of them in Africa, predominantly among the under-fives (Figure 14.1). The WHO has a target to halve deaths from malaria by 2010, but increasing resistance to malarial drugs makes it unlikely that the target will be achieved. New drugs are expensive and difficult to produce.

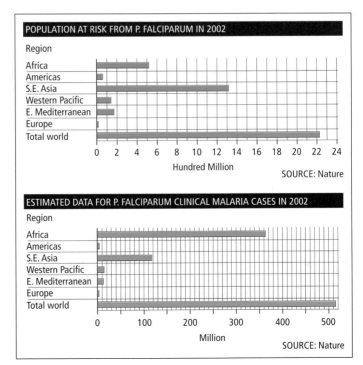

Figure 14.1 Populations at risk and clinical cases of *falciparum* malaria in 2002 (Adapted by permission from Macmillan Publishers Ltd: *Nature*, © 2005).

Malaria has been eradicated from certain parts of the world, such as southern Europe, but has been resurgent elsewhere. The reasons for this include:

- Loss of or reduction in vector control (mosquito) programmes.
- Growing resistance of the mosquito vector to insecticides.
- Growing resistance of the parasite to cheap and common anti-malarial drugs.
- Expansion of irrigated land and areas of standing water (mosquito breeding grounds).

While malaria is not endemic in the UK, globalization means that between 1500 and 2000 cases occur every year in travellers returning to the UK from malaria-endemic countries. Approximately three-quarters of these are caused by *Plasmodium falciparum*, which is responsible for between 10 and 20 deaths in the UK annually. Most patients with *falciparum* malaria acquire their infection in Africa, with West Africa the commonest geographical source.

Factors affecting the risk of being bitten by a malaria-carrying mosquito in a malarial area include temperature, altitude and season, traveller activities, length of stay and methods of travel. Prevalence is generally higher in rural than in urban areas, but it is possible to acquire the disease in cities too. Bite prevention is the first line of defence. Outdoor activities between dusk and dawn, when mosquito activity is at its height, carry a high risk, and backpackers have a higher risk of being bitten compared with tourists staying in air-conditioned hotels and travelling in air-conditioned buses.

Two-thirds of malaria cases in the UK occur in people of African or South Asian ethnic origin and over half of the cases occur in those who have been visiting friends and relatives (VFRs) in endemic areas. They tend to travel to malarial areas more frequently than other travellers and are less likely to take anti-malarial prophylaxis. There tends to be a perception among this group that malaria is a relatively trivial disease and that those born in malarial areas have immunity to it. Both perceptions have been described as 'dangerous myths'. Malaria can be very serious and any

immunity acquired through earlier exposure is quickly lost after migration to the UK. Nor do second-generation migrants (the children of migrants) have any clinically relevant immunity: children under 16 are over-represented in incidence figures for malaria, accounting for 14% of cases. Furthermore, an acute attack of malaria does not confer protection from future attacks: individuals who have had malaria still need to take effective anti-mosquito precautions and chemical prophylaxis during subsequent visits to endemic areas. VFRs form a particular target group for health education work prior to travel.

The Advisory Committee on Malaria Prevention in UK Travellers (ACMP) produces annual guidelines for health professionals advising travellers from the UK. While caution is important, there is also a need for accurate geographical knowledge of the distribution of malaria in overseas countries so that those who are unlikely to contract it can decide accordingly whether prophylaxis is worthwhile. Table 14.1 shows ACMP advice on chemoprophylaxis in South Asia, which highlights the importance of knowing the specific destinations that travellers to this region will be visiting.

Health care needs of asylum seekers

Refugees and asylum seekers to the UK represent a category of people with distinct health care needs. Annual numbers of asylum seekers fluctuate depending on the international political situation and changes to government policy and practice (Figure 14.2). Asylum seekers are not a homogeneous group: in 2006 the top five nations seeking asylum were Eritrea, Afghanistan, China, Iran and Somalia. The prior experience and health care needs of these different nationalities can vary considerably, as can the specific needs of men, women, children and the elderly within them. In 2006, 55% of all principal asylum seekers were males aged between 15 and 34.

Asylum seekers will be granted refugee status if they meet the definition of a refugee set by a 1951 UN convention, namely someone with a 'well founded fear of persecution on the grounds of

Table 14.1 ACMP advice on malaria chemoprophylaxis in South Asia (source: Swales et al, *Journal of Infection*).

Risk	Country	ACMP-recommended regimen	Alternative regimen if recommended regimen unsuitable
Risk high Chloroquine resistance high	*Bangladesh* (only in Chittagong Hill Tract Districts) *India* (Assam)	Mefloquine OR Doxycycline OR Atovaquone/Proguanil	Chloroquine plus Proguanil
Risk variable Chloroquine resistance usually moderate	*Bhutan* (southern districts only) *India* (except for Assam where high risk, and for areas listed below where low risk) *Nepal* (below 1500 m, especially Terai Districts; no risk in Kathmandu) *Pakistan* (below 2000 m) *Sri Lanka* (risk north of Vavuniya)	Chloroquine plus Proguanil	Mefloquine OR Doxycycline OR Atovaquone/Proguanil
Risk low	*Bangladesh* (except Chittagong Hill Tracts, see above) *India* (low risk in southern states of Kerala; Tamil Nadu; Karnataka; Goa and Southern Andhra Pradesh including Hyderabad and the city of Mumbai (Bombay). Low to no risk in northern states of Rajasthan; Uttar Pradesh; Haryana; Punjab; Delhi; Uttaranchal; Himachal Pradesh; Jammu and Kashmir) For other areas see above *Sri Lanka* (low risk in all areas except north of Vavuniya, see above)	Awareness of small risk of malaria; avoid mosquito bites and seek medical attention for any suspicious symptoms (up to about a year later) but tablets not considered necessary	

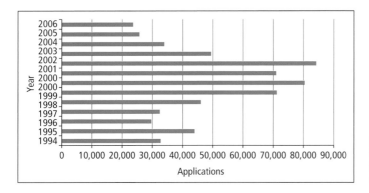

Figure 14.2 Asylum applications to the UK by year. (Source: National Statistics website, www.statistics.gov. uk)

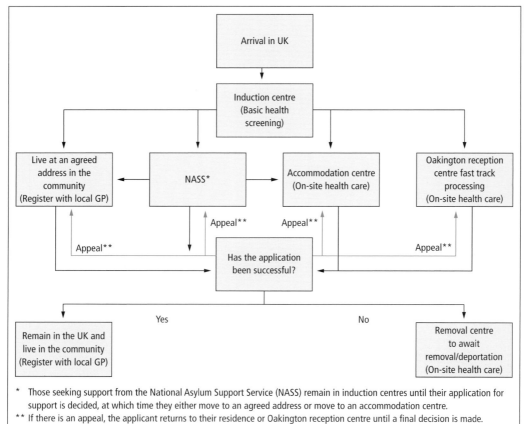

* Those seeking support from the National Asylum Support Service (NASS) remain in induction centres until their application for support is decided, at which time they either move to an agreed address or move to an accommodation centre.

** If there is an appeal, the applicant returns to their residence or Oakington reception centre until a final decision is made.

Figure 14.3 The immigration process for asylum seekers in the UK, with associated health care services (Source: British Medical Association 2002).

race, religion, nationality, membership of a particular social group or political opinion'. The process of gaining asylum is a tortuous one involving four stages (see Figure 14.3). Since 2002, all

people claiming asylum on arrival in the UK are taken to an induction centre where they are held for between one and seven days, after which they are either moved to an agreed address or, if they need accommodation, to an accommodation centre or the fast track (7–10 day) processing centre at Oakington, in Cambridgeshire. Applicants are interviewed about their history of persecution and right to remain in the UK and have to present evidence to substantiate their claim. The Home Office aims to decide on each case within two months. Only about 25% of asylum seekers have their applications upheld, either as refugees or as people granted 'exceptional leave to remain'. Appeals are expected to be decided on in the courts within four months.

It is estimated that there are 280,000 people living in Britain having had their application refused. Many are destitute although they prefer to remain in the country illegally rather than return home where they might face torture or being killed.

Health problems of asylum seekers

Likely health problems and contributory factors experienced by asylum seekers and refugees include:

Communicable diseases	**Psychological and social health problems**
• Tuberculosis	• Depression
• Hepatitis A, B and/or C	• Anxiety
• HIV/AIDS	• Stress
• Parasitic infections	• Stress-related physical ill health:
	○ Heart disease
Effects of war and torture	○ Cancer
• Landmine injuries	○ Increased susceptibility to infection
• Amputated limbs	○ Gastrointestinal disturbances
• Lameness	• 'Fear syndrome' or fear of people in authority
• Partial loss of vision	• Deprivation of human rights
• Hearing difficulties	• Political repression
• Mental health problems	• Harassment/racial harassment
(see next column)	• Loss of status
• Injuries arising from beatings and torture (including	• Homesickness
dental torture)	• Separation from family
• Rape/sexual assault	• Change in climate
• Malnutrition (could affect development in children)	• Uncertainty around the process of claiming
• Lack of personal protection	asylum in the UK
• Conscription into the army (adults and children)	• Lack of awareness about available services
• Prolonged squalor in camps	• Coping with new culture/limited or no access
• Detention	to community network
• Witnessing death and torture of others	
• Held under siege	
• Forcible destruction of home or property	
• Disappearance of family/friends	
• Held hostage or as human shield	

The threats to asylum seekers' and refugees' health are mostly those of communicable, degenerative and psychological diseases linked to poverty and overcrowding, and are not specific to their refugee status, although this status may make them particularly acute. Asylum seekers are socially excluded and vulnerable to poor health.

Many of the health problems they face are common to all deprived and excluded groups. Others are more specific to them, and may originate from physical or mental torture, or other harsh conditions from which they have escaped or have experienced during their journey to the UK (such as those who are smuggled into the country illegally by human traffickers). Many may be separated from their families and face considerable psychological and emotional uncertainty about their claim to asylum. They can feel cultural bereavement from their place of origin and alienation in the UK. Asylum seekers are frequently from fairly affluent backgrounds in their countries of origin, but their children's education may well have been disrupted. All these things add to the likelihood of their experiencing health problems.

One in six refugees is likely to have significant physical health problems restricting their activity, slightly more than the UK average. However, a far greater proportion (about two-thirds) will have experienced significant anxiety or depression. The government's policy of dispersing asylum seekers away from the pressure points of London and the South East leads to further stress and strain due to isolation, reduced social support, poor quality accommodation, and hostility and prejudice from the community they are moved into. Dietary habits are also likely to differ markedly from those of the host communities. Many have difficulty finding familiar foods at reasonable prices and lack adequate food preparation and storage facilities in their accommodation.

Providing health care for asylum seekers

Asylum seekers are entitled to primary and secondary health care without charge. Failed asylum seekers who are not appealing their decision are not eligible for free secondary health care, although the Department of Health has agreed that any hospital treatment already underway when their claim is rejected should continue free of charge until clinical judgement is that it has been completed. Primary health care provision for failed asylum seekers is at time of writing under review and is very much at the discretion of individual GP practices, although emergency and immediately necessary treatment is provided free of charge to anyone, again dependent on the clinical opinion of the doctor that it is required. Primary care groups in areas to which many asylum seekers are dispersed sometimes set up primary care units dedicated to the specific needs of asylum seekers.

As a group, asylum seekers may have particular problems in health care settings. For example, the concept of screening may be alien, since screening might have been unavailable or of very restricted availability in their countries of origin. Their prior experiences (such as rape) may make having what would be a routine investigation such as cervical screening very difficult. Clitoridectomy (female genital mutilation) is a cultural practice that is particularly common in Eritrea and Somalia (two of the primary asylum seeker origin nations at the present time) which also poses potential problems for doctors working with women from these countries. The language/culture barrier that many have is common to others from ethnic minorities who do not speak English (see Chapter 8) and is exacerbated by relatively recent arrival in the UK and the 'culture shock' that goes with it. Asylum seekers often have other demands on their time – they may be going to college, have appointments with solicitors, need to look after their children or be living at some distance from their health care without good knowledge of public transport links. Furthermore, the high incidence of reactive depression and distress may make it harder for patients to motivate themselves to access health care at all. Another issue faced by doctors working with asylum seekers is the extreme mobility of the population and the likelihood of a patient moving (or being moved) at short notice. This can make follow-up appointments or treatment difficult to organize.

Points of view: HIV/AIDS testing in recent immigrants and asylum seekers: opt-in or opt-out?

Around one third of those infected with HIV in the UK at any time are currently undiagnosed. The asylum seeker/recent immigrant population not only currently makes up the largest group of new diagnoses of HIV infection (about half of all diagnoses in 2006); they are also the group with the largest number of undiagnosed HIV infections. Failure to diagnose early results in patients presenting late (with AIDS), often with high mortality and an increased risk of the disease being transmitted to others.

The traditional way of running HIV screening services in the UK has been an 'opt-in' system. This is where patients are introduced to the idea of an HIV test, are advised or encouraged to have one, and are then asked if they want to have one. There is pre-test counselling and consent is formally given. However, uptake of HIV screening through the 'opt-in' system is dependent on a number of factors:

- It being offered in the first place (a study of HIV-positive African men in London found that 80% reported not having been offered a test during visits to GP surgeries)
- The persuasiveness of the health professional (who may have a legitimate concern for patient autonomy and 'right to choose')
- The attitude of the patient to the idea of being tested (since HIV is still a highly stigmatized condition and many regard a positive diagnosis as a death sentence).

For these reasons, there has recently been discussion about moving to an 'opt-out' system whereby, patients would be told that they were going to have a set of routine blood tests, one of which would include HIV, and asked whether they had any questions. There would only be pre-test counselling about the test at the doctor's discretion if she or he felt there was a significant risk of the patient being HIV-positive. Consent would not be formally given. The assumption is that universal 'opt-out' testing will yield a larger number of tests and a greater percentage detection rate. As such it has been recommended by the WHO and United Nations AIDS Committee.

Opt-out HIV screening has been standard practice in antenatal care in the UK for almost a decade, with the benefit of substantially reducing mother-to-child transmission by picking up undiagnosed infections, as well as identifying more HIV-infected women. It is also becoming the preferred testing strategy in genitourinary medicine (GUM) clinics. It is regarded as a cost-effective option for all countries with a prevalence rate of HIV of 0.2% or more, and a recent Standards for HIV Clinical Care document recommends moving towards an opt-out strategy for HIV testing in 'all relevant clinical settings' in the UK.

Unlike in some countries, HIV testing is not manadatory for immigrants and asylum seekers entering the UK. In the past, HIV was effectively an untreatable illness, and hence testing was a considerable emotional strain. However, the advent of anti-retroviral drug therapy in the last decade has offered an effective form of treatment and has turned what was commonly regarded as a 'death sentence' into a treatable disease with much the same status as diabetes (although only if it is detected in good time). In this context, an 'opt-out' system appears to make sense. Some countries such as Botswana have adopted it for the general population and acceptance has been good. In the case of asylum seekers, patients may want assurance that their test result will have no bearing on the outcome of their case. The likelihood is that most health care facilities will use some kind of hybrid system, with (say) a patient from a country known to have a high prevalence of HIV being given extra encouragement to have a test, or a patient being given pre-test counselling prior to a routine test.

The recent developments of HIV rapid testing kits, which give results within seconds, raise new issues concerning pre- and post-test counselling and consent.

Medical tourism

The movement of wealthy people for theraputic purposes is nothing new – travel to the seaside or to spa towns for one's health are both well-known traditions in the UK. However, in recent years the ease and relative cheapness of long-distance travel has led to more and more people taking advantage of cheaper health care costs abroad and seeking out what is effectively cut-price private health care overseas. Not all health problems can be exported in this way. The degree of urgency of a health problem tends to downgrade its exportability, with acute infectious diseases unlikely to be taken abroad for treatment, but services such as opthalmology, orthopaedics and dentistry, preventive services (check-ups) and cosmetic surgery are more likely to be exported. Triggers to travelling abroad for health care include cost of treatment, waiting times in the home country, and the attractiveness of combining such a venture with an overseas holiday (Figure 14.4). Sometimes the impetus to travel will not come from the individual, but from a trend in outsourcing health care from nations with overstretched health services to countries where there is spare capacity. There are also increasing numbers of wealthy people from poorer countries such as Bangladesh travelling abroad to secure health care that is unavailable at home.

Certain countries are putting a great deal of effort and resources into promoting medical tourism and are developing niche markets and targeting particular sectors (Figure 14.5). The Indian government, for example, calculated its foreign currency earnings from its 150,000 medical tourists in 2004 as approximately £180 million, and anticipates this will grow at a rate of 30% a year. It has been calculated that medical tourism worldwide in 2010 will be a £20 billion business with 780 million people seeking some form of health care outside their normal country of residence.

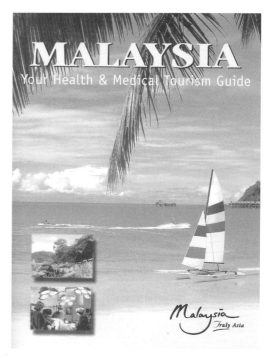

Figure 14.4 Cover of a Malaysian health tourism brochure.

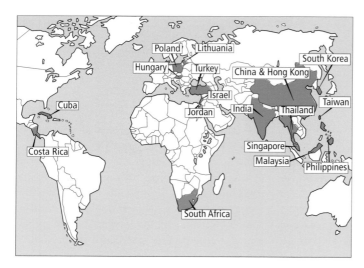

Figure 14.5 Some of the most active countries in the field of health tourism, 2007.

A patient comes to their GP with a plan to travel overseas for medical treatment. What are the pitfalls the doctor should outline?

- The costs can be high and have to be met from the patient's own pocket.
- Language barriers can make it difficult for the patient to communicate their needs.
- Opportunities for follow-up care are limited. The patient usually only spends a few days in hospital or receiving treatment, after which they may have a holiday in the country or return home immediately. Complications and side-effects and post-operative care are difficult to manage in these circumstances and may become the responsibility of the health care system at home.
- Most of the countries offering medical tourism have weaker malpractice laws than the UK, so if something goes wrong the patient has little redress.
- There is a moral argument that private sector organizations engaged in medical tourism are drawing medical resources and personnel away from serving the local populace. Some medical organizations are starting to provide a local service as well, however (e.g. by making a quota of beds available to local people free of charge).

The risk of global pandemics

Despite the increase in chronic illness (see Chapter 12) infectious diseases still account for a third of all deaths worldwide (half of those in developing countries, one in seven of those in developed countries). Most novel infections of recent years have been zoonoses (infections transmitted from vertebrates to humans). The risk of zoonotic diseases may be increasing with the encroachment of human habitation into animal habitats and increasing densities of both human and livestock populations worldwide (Table 14.2). The major public health risk from zoonotic infections is if they mutate and become transmissible from person to person. If this happens, it can cause a pandemic (an epidemic of a new disease affecting a large area of the globe) because of lack of immunity in the general population. The UK may be particularly at risk of human–human zoonotic infection as it is one of the most globally well connected countries, and is relatively small for its size and density of population.

In 2003, SARS came close to causing a pandemic from a souce in South East Asia. At its height, 120 million people in the region were quarantined to prevent its spread. HIV is much slower in its spread due to its non-airborne mode of transmission.

In order to prevent pandemics, it is necessary to detect unexplained clusters of possible infectious diseases. Standard surveillance measures are traditionally poor at cluster detection. The Global Public Health Intelligence Network (GPHIN), introduced in 1997, is a search engine based in Canada that continuously scans open websites, in seven languages, for reports of unexplained illnesses in over 950 local media sources around

Table 14.2 Examples of zoonoses which have become capable of human-human transmission in the past 50 years.

Zoonotic disease	Original source (speculative)
Avian influenza (e.g. H5N1 virus)	Poultry populations in South East Asia
Bovine Spongiform Encephalopathy (BSE) (known as Creutzfeldt Jakob disease in its human form)	Ruminant animals
Ebola and Marburg viruses	Bats in Africa?
Severe Acute Respiratory Syndrome (SARS)	Civet cats in China?
HIV	Simian populations in Africa

the world. On average, 18,000 items are picked up every day, of which around 200 merit further analysis by WHO. Over the past ten years, 40–50% of initial alerts to outbreaks, subsequently investigated by WHO, came from the media and other non-official sources. SARS was indicated as a health problem in south China in 2002 before it spread to Hong Kong in 2003, while H5N1 infections in ducks in China were detected in 2004. This useful tool is being developed further.

Once a disease is spreading from person-to-person contact, a chain reaction means it spreads exponentially. Such growth stops only when the disease begins to run out of new people to infect, or falls to below replacement levels and hence goes into decline. At this point, it has become endemic and the disease reaches equilibrium.

Ways of reducing epidemic transmission

Method	Examples
Reduce contact	Individual and household quarantine; social distancing (e.g. school closures)
Reduce susceptibility	Vaccination; antiviral prophylaxis
Reduce infectiousness	Antiviral treatment; infection control measures (e.g. wearing surgical masks)

The key issues in reducing transmission are who is targeted, how much effort is required and how fast one has to act. Mathematical modelling is helpful at quantifying the degree of risk or uncertainty.

Case study: Avian influenza – a major global public health priority

Influenza is a bird virus of many strains – most waterfowl have been infected at least once in their lives, usually with a virus of the digestive tract that is of low pathogenicity. Avian influenza or 'bird flu' characteristically arises from a more highly pathogenic virus. One strain of many dozens is H5N1 virus, which is currently giving particular cause for concern because of its high mortality rate in humans (currently greater than 50%). This compares with a maximum mortality rate of 10% in the 1918 influenza epidemic. However, it has proved to be poor at jumping from birds to humans, and – so far – very limited in its ability to spread from person to person.

It has been calculated that were H5N1 to become as contagious as normal human influenza, an epidemic of H5N1 in the UK would peak at 50 days after the first case and would be likely to cause 15% absenteeism. As the incubation period for influenza is short – 1–2 days – and people are at their most infectious very soon after symptoms appear, transmission is very rapid (doubling in two days; a tenfold increase in 7–14 days). Thus it is necessary to be able to detect an outbreak at fewer than 50 cases, and to react to all new cases within two days. Containment of H5N1 virus would need intensive quarantining measures and blanket use of antivirals, not ony to reduce symptoms and infectiousness but also as prophylaxis for the uninfected. The value of travel restrictions is less clear. Given the transmissibility statistic, it can be calculated that stopping 90% of infections would only buy 1–2 weeks' time; stopping 99% of infections would gain 2–4 weeks' time. School closure would also delay transmission somewhat. Vaccines can take six months to produce so stockpiling in advance is necessary. Masks are of uncertain benefit, although France has stockpiled one million as part of its health protection preparations.

Whatever happens, if the population can survive the first wave of infection, it is likely that HP51 virus will become endemic and less lethal to the community. We are still living with the H1N1 virus in our midst which killed 40–50 million people worldwide in 1918. Two subsequent but far less catastrophic influenza pandemics have occurred since then – one in 1957 and one in 1968.

Globalization and its effects on health and health care in poor countries

Globalization offers opportunities for multi-country and multi-regional initiatives in health, some of which have been very successful. The eradication of smallpox and the near-eradication of poliomyelitis during the twentieth century are success stories that could only have been accomplished in a globalized world. Some aspects of globalization, such as economic growth and the spread of new technologies, have also been beneficial for health and have increased overall life expectancy, at least in the short term. Some notable exceptions to this trend exist, however. Countries in the former Soviet Union, such as Belarus, Ukraine, Kazakhstan and the Russian Federation itself, experienced a decline in life expectancy in the 1990s as economic liberalization led to sharp increases in unemployment, growing disparities of wealth and the breakdown of the social support mechanisms of communism. The excess of deaths during this period has been estimated at four million. Other aspects of globalization may be putting health in jeopardy in the long term through their negative influence on social and environmental conditions.

Globalization affects the following determinants of health in poor countries:

- Income and income distribution.
- Health services and systems.
- Global institutions.
- The wider health context.

Income and income distribution

The links between income and health are well known, with rising income among poor people leading to improved nutrition, better child survival rates, improved maternal health and higher levels of female education, all of which are associated with or contribute further to positive health outcomes. Many economists have assumed that an open trade and investment policy will accelerate income generation in poor countries. However, this is not a universally true.

Prerequisites for open trade and investment policies to accelerate income growth in poor countries

- Non-exclusionary markets (i.e. no or few import barriers imposed by other countries).
- Strong national fiscal and regulatory institutions.
- Some kind of social contract offering a safety net when things go wrong (e.g. companies or markets fail).
- Good human and physical infrastructure.

Countries which have these characteristics and have demonstrated impressive health gains over the past 20 or so years include China, Costa Rica, the East Asian 'tiger economies' and Vietnam.

For many countries in Africa, Latin America and Eastern Europe, however, poor domestic conditions, unequal distribution of foreign investments and the imposition of conditions limiting the access of their exports to the markets of richer nations has meant that growth has been slow, unstable or nonexistent, poverty has increased and health indicators have been stagnant or have fallen. It is unlikely that further market liberalization will help them improve their economies or the health status of their citizens. The removal of asymmetric relationships in global markets, the creation of more democratic institutions and public sector development and reform are likely to be more effective at improving health than increasingly unfettered globalization – there is no 'global social contract' when globalization fails.

Health services and health systems

Effective health systems not only cure people, but also, if design and management incorporate preventive as well as curative measures, reduce the financial costs of illness to the individual and to society as a whole, contribute to a sense of social cohesion and help to allay anxieties about vulnerability and powerlessness which are central to the experience of poverty. Hundreds of millions of people worldwide still lack access to even basic health care, and where they do, such care frequently has to be paid for, so pushing already poor people into destitution. Approximately £6 billion in health sector aid is given annually by richer countries to poorer ones. By comparison, a similar amount is spent on ice cream in Europe every year and about ten times this amount goes on the NHS budget in England. Much of the health sector aid that is given is uncoordinated and focused on specific diseases rather than assisting the development of the health system as a whole. In addition, structural adjustment programmes (see below) and their accompanying compulsory economic reforms often lead to the further commercialization of health care and reduced availability of

the public services which are most used by poor people. Higher levels of private finance and commercial health provision have been shown to lead to worse health outcomes: widening health care inequities, more limited access to quality care for the poor as public systems become sidelined, greater duplication of effort and other inefficiencies, and a breakdown in trust and ethical behaviour. Many countries (not just poor ones) need support and encouragement to build universal health systems that are financed by taxation or affordable private insurance.

Globalization has the potential to undermine the quality of health services and systems in poor countries. This section considers two ways in which this can happen: the 'brain drain' of health professionals from poor countries, and the role of the pharmaceutical industry.

Migrating doctors: a global health issue

One of the ways in which globalization has had a direct effect on health and health care is in the mobility of doctors and other health professionals who can now migrate between countries. The concern is that this migration is largely one way – from poor, developing countries to rich, developed ones. In this way poorer countries, which have borne the cost of educating and training the doctors, are subsidizing the developed countries, which reap the benefit from their skills. Furthermore, the migration of doctors and nurses can leave the poorer countries, which in public health terms have greater health needs, with severe staff shortages. Some developed countries, including Britain, have actively recruited health professionals from developing countries as a solution to perceived national shortages. Low pay, poor conditions and limited career opportunities – even unemployment in some cases – are potent forces pushing doctors from resource-poor countries towards the UK. For the UK, international recruitment provides a 'quick fix' to deal with staff shortages, since it takes at least ten years to train a 'home-grown' doctor from scratch.

In 2002, registration data from the General Medical Council showed that nearly half of the 10,000 new doctors on the register were from overseas; in 2003 this risen to more than two-thirds of the total (15,000). Most of these overseas entrants were from countries outside the European Economic Area. This situation is paralleled in other parts of the developed world: 24% of the US medical workforce were essentially trained free of charge to the US, while in Australia roughly 20% of the workforce has been actively recruited from overseas, primarily to fill positions in rural areas.

There are two policy options for dealing with these problems: a *laissez-faire* approach; or management intervention involving bilateral agreements between countries, staff exchanges or regional initiatives to manage the migration process. The Department of Health has issued a code of practice requiring NHS employers to avoid recruiting actively from developing countries, unless an agreement between the two governments has been made. However, in 2003, one in three nurse work permits issued were to applicants who came from these developing countries, mainly in sub-Saharan Africa.

This 'skills drain' can have a very negative impact on the health systems of the countries these health professionals leave. It is argued by some that poorer countries should be paid full compensation by the richer countries that poach their staff. The migration of health professionals has become an important debate in international health policy circles

Arguments for and against the migration of doctors

For	Against
• Doctors should have the right to do what they like, whether it is moving or staying.	• Doctors have an obligation to serve the needs of the nation in which they trained.
• The figures for costs are flawed. Not all doctors will have trained at the taxpayers' expense. They still have to take qualifying examinations at their own expense once they arrive, and pay tax to the host country like every other professional.	• The cost of training the doctors is borne by the country of origin and their migration represents a net wealth transfer from the poorer to richer countries without any recompense.
• Migration is a symptom of deeper problems in some health systems – planning failure, low pay, lack of career prospects. These issues need to be addressed nationally and internationally, then the migration issue would solve itself.	• The broader issues of health development in a poor country are complex, but cannot be resolved if the haemorrhage of its brightest and best doctors is allowed to continue.
• Doctors have a right to aspire to a lucrative salary and urban lifestyle like everybody else. They may have debts to clear and families to support.	• Doctoring is a vocation and money should not be the 'be all and end all' of a doctor's motivation; serving the needs of others should be paramount.
• There can be benefits to the poorer countries in migration of health professionals overseas – through remittances back home, development of skills and experience of other organizational systems	• Migrants are unlikely to return to their countries of origin, therefore any skills developed will not be deployed 'back home' (assuming the home countries provide the facilities and resources to deploy these skills). Nor will migrants necessarily send remittances.
• Interventions and rules to manage the migration of health professionals are largely untested and are unlikely to work.	• Interventions and rules are required to deal with the problem so that doctors are only recruited from appropriate countries.

Overall it seems the debate on the migration of doctors and other health professionals needs to shift from concern over numbers (how many?) to concern about what effective approaches there might be for managing and moderating the process (how?), assuming this is necessary. More focus on social development issues in medical education would help develop the social conscience of trainees and make them more likely to develop careers that reflected this. Some countries have requirements that every graduate spends a period of time working in rural or other underserved areas. Migration of health care workers cannot be addressed by individual countries in isolation. If regulation is necessary, it should be part of a wider strategy to improve the health services of both poorer and richer countries. But the power structures inherent in international relations mean that negotiations at the global level will not take place on a level playing field.

The movement of medicines

The 'magic bullet' approach to illness, which is often sought by patients and promulgated by the health industry as part of the medicalization of society (Chapter 1), means potentially huge profits for the companies that manufacture pharmaceutical products (see below). The free distribution of medicinal drugs between nations with very different regulatory frameworks means that drugs can be used in very different ways in poorer countries. Inadequate packaging and instructions that are not printed in locally understood languages mean that drugs may used in ways very different from those the manufacturers intended or recommend. Drugs that are only available on prescription in the Anglo-American world, for example, may be purchasable on an 'over-the-counter' basis in a general store in a poor country, or may be distributed by a folk sector practitioner such as the mobile 'injection doctor'.

Advantages and disadvantages of having pharmaceuticals available in an under-regulated way in poorer countries

Advantages	Disadvantages
• They can be distributed widely, helping to alleviate symptoms and treat common conditions even in areas where other sources of health care may be lacking.	• Contributes to increasing medicalization of illness with emphasis on drug treatment only.
• People can buy what they want when they want.	• There can be serious problems with side-effects, allergies, deliberate and inadvertent overdosing.
• Local pharmacists can provide advice and information, as well as medicines, more cheaply and easily than a doctor.	• Local pharmacists and other practitioners may be unqualified and sometimes even illiterate. Sometimes they can charge more than qualified health personnel.
• Those with stigmatized conditions can purchase treatment anonymously.	• Drugs can be used inappropriately (e.g. viral infections treated with antibiotics).
• Many of the problems in the 'disadvantages' column are found among users of prescription drugs in richer countries too – it's not a rich/poor country issue.	• Often people on antibiotics cut corners by only using a few tablets when they should complete a full course, hence enabling the development of drug-resistant strains of infection such as TB to evolve.
	• Sometimes drugs can be out of date and hence ineffective; counterfeit drugs are also a big problem.

Case Study: the WHO's Essential Drugs and Medicines Programme

The WHO's Essential Drugs and Medicines Programme was established in 1977 with the aim of 'closing the huge gap between the potential that essential drugs have to offer and the reality that for millions of people – particularly the poor and disadvantaged – medicines are unavailable, unaffordable, unsafely used'. The programme is based on the principle of agreeing clinical guidelines to decide at the national level about a limited number of carefully selected and vetted medicines being made available.

• Within the context of a functioning health system.
• At all times.
• In adequate amounts.
• In appropriate dosage forms.
• With assured quality and adequate information.
• At a price that individuals and communities can afford.

The programme was intended to lead to more rational prescribing practices, a better supply of medicines and lower costs, in order to save lives and improve health. Countries would produce their own national essential medicines lists and drug formularies which became the basis of formal education and training of health professionals and of health education for the general public about appropriate medicine use. These lists would also serve as the basis for public sector drug procurement and distribution, preferably using locally produced versions or generic forms bulk-purchased from the pharmaceutical companies. They were also intended to guide decision-making regarding drug donations, to prevent the practice of dumping of surplus and superfluous pharmaceuticals by drug companies which was a problem for poorer countries. There are over 250 medicines listed on the WHO's 15th 'Model List of Essential Drugs', a document that has been updated every two years since 1977.

Opposition to the notion of an essential drugs list has come not only from sections of the pharmaceutical industry but sometimes from local people who are attracted to the more expensively packaged, imported brand name drugs rather than to the locally produced alternatives. The danger is that too much focus on drug treatments will encourage the belief that health enhancement derives from consuming expensive medicines rather than improving living conditions.

Global institutions

This section focuses on the World Bank and the International Monetary Fund (IMF) as two key global institutions that have a powerful influence on global health. Public services around the world have been affected by constraints put on public expenditure through the structural adjustment programmes instituted by the World Bank and the IMF in exchange for funds to keep the faltering economies of poor countries afloat. These two institutions are now the dominant force in terms of aid and development worldwide, but are criticized for being undemocratic and imposing conditions on poor countries that adversely affect the health of their most vulnerable citizens.

Both institutions are based in Washington, DC and are interlinked. The World Bank is not a bank in the conventional sense, but acts like a fund, lending money for development projects. The IMF, by contrast, is a fund that acts like a bank, providing temporary financial help to countries that have difficulties with their balance of payments. Countries join the IMF by depositing a quota subscription that determines both how much they can withdraw in a crisis, and their voting rights in both institutions. Typical borrowing periods are 1–4 years with repayments expected in 3–10 years. Loans come, however, at the cost of dictated short-term macroeconomic and fiscal measures to restore a country's financial health. Loans are disbursed in instalments to ensure these reforms take place.

A country must be a member of the IMF if it wishes to borrow from the World Bank. The World Bank's mission is to reduce global poverty and increase living standards. It currently lends about £10 billion a year for this purpose. It does so through two linked development institutions: the International Bank for Reconstruction and Development (IBRD) and the International Development Association (IDA). The former provides loans, credit and grants to middle-income and creditworthy poor countries (primarily using money generated by the sale of bonds to private investors), while the IDA does the same with interest-free loans and grants to the poorest countries (using monies raised from the richer countries every three years). Bank economists rank the policy performance of low-income countries to determine the amount of lending they may receive.

The World Bank began by granting loans for specific projects – usually infrastructural development such as road construction, dams and telecommunications services. However, corruption, poor project design and management and sharp increases in interest rates put many developing countries into deep debt with the Bank. Thus in 1980, the Bank became more like the IMF in starting to give long-term loans to deal with recurrent balance of payments problems, but linked these to stringent structural adjustment programmes (SAPs).

SAPs were accompanied by a number of conditions. These might include:
- Reducing public expenditure.
- Liberalizing trade, investment and capital controls.
- Privatizing state-owned enterprises.

Agreeing to these requirements enabled the countries concerned to obtain the foreign currency reserves they needed in order to repay their loans. However, the impact of the economic reforms that accompanied restructuring and debt servicing on the health and well-being of poor people was often severe, marked by:
- Rising unemployment.
- Fall in real wages.
- Promotion of the cash crop sector.
- Removal of food subsidies.
- Increase in occupations with health risks (e.g. prostitution).
- Reduction in expenditure on public sector education and health care.
- Cost-recovery strategies introduced for education and health care (e.g. privatization and/or user fees) with consequent fall in utilization.

So unpopular were SAPs and damaging to the Bank's image as a source of development aid that, in 2000, they were renamed Poverty Reduction Support Credits in order to try to emphasize the recipient countries' ownership of the programmes. Governments were expected to write their own

Poverty Reduction Strategy Papers, but these have proved surprisingly similar in their scope to the policies associated with the much hated SAPs.

The World Bank has also been criticized for the types of development project it favours. Many of its infrastructural projects have had negative social and environmental consequences. Large, Bank-funded hydroelectric dam projects, for example, have led to the displacement of indigenous peoples without proper compensation and the destruction of fragile ecosystems. Oil, gas and mining projects, and the pollution of air, land and water associated with them, also give cause for concern, since they seldom seem to lift local people out of poverty.

The wider health context

The 1978 Alma Ata Declaration that there would be 'Health for All by the Year 2000' recognized that achieving this goal required more than improvement to health services. Food, education and clean water were acknowledged as the cornerstones to improving health worldwide. The failure of the Declaration to achieve these goals reflects the broader failure of governments to effect change regionally, nationally and internationally.

In addition to the 'basic needs' of peoples, many of the development policies intended to improve standards of living through agricultural development or industrialization can have unintended side-effects on health. New occupational health risks may emerge, there may be exposure to toxic substances, effluent, radiation, traffic pollution and general environmental degradation. Some of these broader links and interconnections are complex and hard to unravel – for example, global environmental change caused by economic development in some countries is leading to climate change and hence drought and economic decline in others. Arms production that benefits employees of manufacturing companies in the developed world causes disruption and devastation to health and health care systems in war-torn areas. Health care professionals such as doctors, even in their training years, can provide leadership in facilitating and promoting action for health in a variety

of different sectors that might not normally be regarded as part of 'health work'. In an increasingly globalized world, the need for medicine to be involved in the wider social problems of humanity has never been stronger.

Summary

- The increasing mobility of people, goods and ideas around the world is known as globalization. It is a powerful force for health change, both good and bad. The increasing interconnectedness of the world and its people means that health problems in one part of the world are now far more likely to be shared in others.
- Travel medicine is an increasingly important branch of western medicine designed to deal with problems in the richer countries associated with greater mobility of people around the world.
- Asylum seekers are an example of a category of people with distinct health care needs that may be difficult to meet in the western context.
- Increasing numbers of people from richer countries are travelling overseas for reasons of 'medical tourism'. Where things go wrong, dealing with complications can burden the health system of the country of origin.
- Modern communications and computer power make it possible to detect and report new outbreaks of zoonotic diseases that have crossed the human–human transmission threshold, but increasing global mobility means that epidemics are likely to spread faster.
- Globalization has had some positive benefits in poorer countries, such as the total eradication of smallpox and the near-eradication of polio.
- Income and income distribution are major determinants of health and the liberalization of market economies has had positive effects in some countries where safeguards to this process are in place. Other countries have seen declines in their health status as a result of globalization.
- The health systems of poorer countries can be markedly affected by globalization, through the 'brain drain' of health professionals from poorer to richer countries, and the under-regulated flow of pharmaceuticals.

- The World Bank and the IMF are global institutions that have had a profound effect on the financial circumstances of poorer countries and consequently the health of their most vulnerable citizens.
- The need for medical involvement in the wider context of health has never been stronger or more important for the future of the world.

Further reading

British Medical Association (2002) *Asylum Seekers: Meeting their Healthcare Needs*. London: British Medical Association.

Buchan, J. (2005) International recruitment of health professionals. *British Medical Journal*, **330**: 210.

Bulletin of the World Health Organization (2001) Special theme issue: Globalization, **79(9)**. http://www.who.int/bulletin/archives/volume79_9/en/index.html.

Gill, G. V. and Beeching, N. (2004) *Lecture Notes on Tropical Medicine*. Oxford: Blackwell

Global Health Watch (2005) Report. http://www.ghwatch.org/2005_report.php.

Health Protection Agency (2006) Migrant health: infectious diseases in non-UK born populations in England, Wales and Northern Ireland. A baseline report. http://www.hpa.org.uk/publications/2006/migrant_health/default.htm.

Janes, C. (2007) Medical gap years abroad. *BMJ Careers*, **335** (10 November): 169–70.

Lee, K. (2003) *Globalization and Health: an Introduction*. London: Palgrave Macmillan.

McMichael, A.J. and Beaglehole, R. (2000) The changing global context of public health. *The Lancet*, **356**: 495–9.

Phillips, D. R. and Verhasselt, Y. (1994) (eds) *Health and Development*. London: Routledge.

Snow, R. W., Guerra, C. A., Noor, A. M., Myint, H. Y. and Hay, S. I. (2005) The global distribution of clinical episodes of *Plasmodium falciparum* malaria. *Nature*, **434(7030)**: 214–17.

Spira, A. M. (2003) Assessment of travellers who return home ill. *The Lancet*, **361**: 1459–69.

Swales, C. A., Chiodini, P. L. and Bannister, B. A. (2007) New guidelines on malaria prevention: a summary. *Journal of Infection*, **54(2)**: 107–10.

WHO (2005) The Bangkok Charter for Health Promotion in a Globalized World. http://www.who.int/healthpromotion/conferences/6gchp/bangkok_charter/en/index.html.

WHO (2007) *Model List of Essential Medicines* (15th edn.). http://www.who.int/medicines/publications/EML15.pdf.

Glossary

Chronic illness etiquette: the customs or rules which govern how people suffering from chronic illness and those meeting them deal with the illness in social situations.

Community care: the policy of providing health care for individuals in their own homes and communities wherever possible, rather than in a long-stay institution or residential establishment.

Compliance/adherence: two terms that refer to following medical advice correctly by a patient.

Concordance: optimizing health gains from the best use of medicines through a shared approach to decision-making in the consultation.

Cultural competency: the ability of individuals to increase their understanding and appreciation of cultural differences and similarities within, among, and between groups.

Cultural stereotyping: the tendency to ascribe and hence perceive common characteristics amongst all those within a group.

Deinstitutionalization: releasing people from institutional care (such as mental hospitals) into other forms of care provision.

Demedicalization: the process of removing problems previously defined as medical problems from the medical domain.

Diagnostic overshadowing: a dominant illness or condition that negatively affects the accuracy of clinicians' judgements about concomitant illness or conditions.

Disease: an organic pathology or abnormality.

Explanatory models: the particular notions about an illness and its treatment that are brought by those involved to the clinical process.

Folk sector: all healers and therapists who are not part of the 'official' medical system.

Globalization: the compression of space and time associated with the greater and increasingly rapid mobility of people, objects and ideas within and between countries around the world.

Health inequalities: the uneven distribution of health and health care within and between communities regions and nations.

Health-seeking behaviour: the ways in which individuals, families, communities and society seek to maintain and improve health and deal with ill health.

Hierarchy of resort: the order in which people decide to use particular forms of therapy.

Humoral system: sees the body as made up of four humours – blood, phlegm, yellow bile and black bile – the balance of which is the basis of good health.

Iatrogenesis: illness that derives from medical treatment.

Illness: the subjective experience of ill health.

Inverse care law: 'the availability of good medical care tends to vary inversely with the need of the population served'.

Labelling: attaching descriptive words to people that influence the attitudes and behaviour of others towards them.

Lay referral networks: the social networks through which individuals pass before seeking professional advice.

Medicalization: the process of defining an increasing number of life's problems as medical problems.

Medical pluralism: the coexistence of a variety of different types of medical system.

Patient-centred care: placing the interests of the patient, his or her ideas, concerns and expectations, at the heart of clinical practice.

Placebo: an inert substance having no discernible pharmacological effect.

Popular sector: the lay, non-professional, non-specialist cultural arena in which most unpaid healthcare activity takes place, mainly within the sufferer's own social network.

Professional sector: all medical and paramedical professionals organized into a legally sanctioned healing system, such as western biomedicine.

Reflective practitioner: someone who pays deliberate, systematic and analytical attention to what they do, with a view to learning from experience and applying this learning to future action.

Self-help groups: groups designed to help those with a condition either through services for individual sufferers and their carers or through lobbying for changes in attitudes or health care provision.

Sickness: the social experience of ill health.

Socialization: the process whereby people and institutions establish a fit with the culture and society of which they are a part.

Somatization: the expression of emotional problems through physical symptoms.

Stigma: negative regard for a condition.

Therapy managing group: group that assembles when someone is sick to take on the role of sifting information, lending support, making decisions and arranging therapeutic options.

Index